A must-read standout in a crowded field of books on food and health. With this book you get more than just the facts you need to regain and maintain an optimized condition of health. What you will understand is the fundamental truth that lies at the core of existence—you create your own reality, inside and out. Take this trip with Toni and she will lead you into the realization that our planet's environmental crisis is a reflection of our own environmental crisis … we are not separate things. This alone is reason enough to read this book.

—Thomas Campbell, physicist, author of *My Big TOE*

A fabulously written book that provides everything we need to know to *significantly* improve our health. From my own experience and studies, I can testify that the information in this book is accurate, well researched, and extremely significant. It provides numerous missing links that are much needed in the Western World today. If everyone in America followed the suggestions in this book, the American people would once again become the healthiest people on Earth.

—Rich Anderson N.D., author of *Cleanse & Purify Thyself*

A captivating and inspiring book into why we must make wiser food choices. Toni has masterfully painted colorful images to help us better understand what creates health and a state of wellbeing for ourselves as well as our planet at large. The wisdom you'll find contained within these many pages took her decades to attain. In following her guidance, you may save your life, the life of someone you love, and the life of our planet. I have dined at Toni's Table and can personally verify that the food she serves is delectably satisfying and will nourish both your body and soul. Thanks, Toni, for putting it all together.

—Michael Ryce, N.D., author of *Why Is This Happening To Me…AGAIN?!*

An interesting and provocative work for those who are constantly striving to find the secrets of health. *EcoDiet* provides us with those secrets and more importantly, provides us with a plan that will assist us in achievir ⋯ I've read hundreds and hundreds of books on health and nutrition and reco   book, "The China Study" to all of my patients. Now next step for those of us who want to integrate these l to-day understanding and routine.

D1361274

—Dave Carpenter, N.D. author of *Change Your Water, Change Your Life*

GET CLEAN GO GREEN

ECODIET

The secrets of an alkaline environment

*Over 100 alkalizing
recipes included*

TONI TONEY

Foreword by Lorne Label, MD, MBA, FAAN

Toni Toney is a *Body Ecologist* who earned her "master's degree" from the highest possible school of learning: *Nature's University*. She is not a medical physician, and as such, this book is a source of information only, and not a substitute for the advice of the reader's personal physician or other any other medical professional, who should be consulted before beginning this or any diet regime or before cleansing and taking any of the recommended herbs or supplements. The *Get Clean Go Green EcoDiet* food, cleansing and supplement program is the one that Toni subscribed to when medicine failed to help her. Her purpose in writing this book is that it might help the reader, too. The author does not subscribe to the readily accepted viewpoint of "disease," but rather views pain and suffering as a body ecology gone out of balance with nature and the natural order of things. She encourages everyone to become a *Body Ecologist* by taking responsibility for the health and sustainability of their own internal environment. This book, *Get Clean Go Green EcoDiet*, is the result of Toni's 25 years experience working as a *Body Ecologist* and Natural Food Chef for clients around the world looking for a more ecologically-balanced, holistic way of living or those who were suffering from what she calls an "ecological breakdown."

All efforts have been made to ensure the accuracy of the information contained in this book as of the date published. The author and the publisher expressly disclaim responsibility for any adverse effects arising from the use or application of the information contained in this book.

Toni's books are spiritual and nutritional in nature and can be purchased from New Earth Publishers. For more information please contact: New Earth Publishers @ 1-877-342-4550 or getcleangogreenecodiet.com.

First paperback edition published 2010

Front jacket design by Eija Strogard
Back jacket design by Sean Keenan
Layout design by Sean Keenan

ISBN 978-0-9827445-0-5

CONTENTS

FOREWORD

Lorne Label, M.D., M.B.A., F.A.A.N.
Associate Clinical Professor of Neurology
David Geffin School of Medicine, UCLA, Los Angeles, CA

This new book, *Get Clean Go Green EcoDiet*, provides a unique and refreshing approach to our health and how it interfaces with the health of our planet. Toni Toney uniquely reveals various interlinking depictions of the human body and the earth and how we are polluting and destroying them both in much the same way. Simultaneously, we are provided an intuitively simple, yet sophisticated approach to both the workings and failings of the ecological world around and within us. And while the thrust of the book is proper nourishment for our bodies, we also learn that ecological balance is what creates health. Imbalance is what creates disease; not just for ourselves but for our planet.

Using both hard and soft science, Toni Toney thoroughly elaborates on the metabolic needs of the human body and the earth we inhabit. She journeys into the health and failures of our body, while comparing and contrasting that with the failing ecology of our planet. She presents an innovative insight to the types of food we feed into our internal atmosphere and how an acid diet loaded with toxic chemicals creates a type of internal acid rain. She then offers an easy-to-follow explanation of the value and procedure involved in measuring the pH of one's urine to see if acid rain is falling within the atmosphere of the body.

We have long known that the earth has been devastated by acid rain and various other pollutants. But up until now, what we haven't known is that the human body has been devastated by this internal acid rain caused by ingesting acid food, acid air, and acid water. The acidic wastes from chemical additives and processed foods may be the common denominator in many degenerative diseases. We know that in many medical conditions, the accumulated acidic waste causes organ damage.

Though still somewhat controversial in the field of medical studies, the information regarding the acid-alkaline balance and its involvement with disease is both intriguing and plausible. The theory behind the alkaline diet is that the human body is alkaline by design, thus our diet should support maintaining a blood pH between 7.35-7.45. Since all foods that we eat, digest, and metabolize produce either an acid or alkaline base (bicarbonate) in the blood, our diet should be alkaline-producing.

In the past, it was questioned whether acid-producing foods actually promotes the loss of essential minerals such as potassium, magnesium, calcium and sodium due to the body trying to restore equilibrium. In the October 2001 *European Journal of Nutrition*, Dr. Katherine Tucker published, *"The Acid-Base Hypothesis: Diet and Bone in the Framingham Osteoporosis Study,"* supporting the role of base-forming foods and nutrients in bone maintenance. More evidence-based studies in this area will be worthwhile. What medical science does know, however, is that certain foods have substantial anti-cancer effects, while others are important in preventing the formation of calcium kidney stones, osteoporosis, and age-related muscle wasting.

This book is much more than just another book on how to eat in an acid-alkaline type fashion. Toni has been teaching her inner ecology dietary principles to students across the world for decades. Finally, she has assimilated her body of knowledge, and described it in a straightforward, easy to follow approach. She explains the reasons why certain foods create a type of environmental SOS signal, a pre-disaster health warning that we must learn to heed the call. There are extensive lists and charts providing exact information of both the best and worst types of food we should or shouldn't be burning for fuel into our internal environment. Proper preparation of these food groups into delicious dishes is another highlight of *Get Clean Go Green EcoDiet*.

In an almost cookbook-type fashion, the first part of *Get Clean Go Green EcoDiet* lays the groundwork for the most ideal diet, both theoretically and practically, that we should all strive for. The second part is the eco-kitchen and cookbook.

Though the U.S. Government's 2005 *Dietary Guidelines for Americans*, entitled, *MyPyramid*, does break down the five food groups: grains, vegetables, fruit, milk, meat and beans, the specifics are vague. There is neither information on the actual contents of each food group nor description of the best and worst of the foods. For example, under the food group *"vegetables,"* the recommendations include "eat more dark green and orange vegetables and dried beans or peas...include fresh, frozen or canned chopped vegetables." The suggestions under the food group "fruit," state "choose a variety of fresh, frozen, canned or dried fruit."

Clearly, the government's recommendations are vague, not helpful, and to some extent, potentially unhealthy. Anyone trying to understand what the best foods to eat and how to prepare them is left stranded. Common sense should tell us that recommending canned fruit with all its sweeteners is not the healthiest approach.

As pointed out in *Get Clean Go Green EcoDiet,* there are large varieties of healthy fruits and vegetables to choose from with surprisingly other types (common to all of us and potentially our favorite foods) that would be best to avoid. The 2005 *MyPyramid* leaves that information unclear. So do many other diet books on the market. Toni Toney clarifies the information for us.

This book is not a panacea. It is a call to action. It will make you think about how the inner environment of the body is a reflection of the outer, which will most likely change your approach to the kind of foods you eat. In fact, I believe it presents one of the easiest guidelines ever to follow in keeping the pH balance correct for excellent health.

Toni Toney's message throughout this book is: We are one. The earth reflects us and we reflect the earth. What is internal to our planet is our internal village. What is external to our planet reflects our external village. Toni says that to shift our planet's environmental crisis around, we need to "be the change" and shift the crisis within ourselves.

I invite you to join us in our crusade for health: a healthy body and a healthy planet. The time is now for each of us to "Answer the Call."

So *Get Clean, Go Green* and enjoy!

Dr. Lorne Label

AUTHOR'S ACKNOWLEDGMENTS

When walking the journey of life, we never walk alone. There are people who join us along the way that influence our lives more than others. There are also experiences we have along the way that influence our tomorrows more than others. Much of what I have learned about food and nutrition did not come from college textbooks or degree programs. It was born out of a real life experience, acquired by my need to understand why I was sick and why medicine failed to help me. Over the years, I have traveled worldwide and studied extensively in search of answers. This book was written from the insights I gleaned regarding how the human body thrives and how it becomes sick and prematurely dies. My gratitude runs deep to all who influenced my path during my search for the truth.

I want to begin by thanking my two children, Bill and Kim, who sparked my driving force toward change. To my daughter-in-law, Halli Toney and son-in-law Josh Horn. To their children and my grandchildren, Camryn, Dayton and Siera.

To Taylor Hay, for introducing me to healthy eating and taking me into my first health food store—Rainbow Blossom in Louisville, Kentucky.

To you who have taught me well.

To the many physicians I worked with throughout the years, the ones who hold to the Hippocratic principles. To Hippocrates, the father of medicine and the greatest physician of his time, who believed in the natural healing process of rest, a good diet, sunlight, fresh air and cleanliness, and taught that there are no patients, only students.

To Dr. Ted Morter, Jr., founder of Morter Health System in Rogers, Arkansas, and creator of the Bio-Energetic Synchronization Technique (BEST), for the various health weekends I attended at your clinic, which changed my life forever and set the foundation for my life's purpose.

To Dr. Thomas Rau, Chief Medical Director of the Paracelsus Clinic in Switzerland and founder of Paracelsus Biological Medicine, for the many insights you shared with me about human health and the biological terrain during my month-long stay at your clinic.

To Dr. Richard Anderson, founder of Arise & Shine and author of *Cleanse & Purify Thyself,* for the knowledge you shared with me throughout the years about cleansing and restoring a healthy pH balance to our intestinal ecology.

To Dr. Michael Ryce, founder of Heartland Teaching and Retreat Center in Theodosia, Missouri and author of *Why Is This Happening To Me, Again,* for the six months I spent at your center attending your classes on how to truly forgive.

To the many editors that evolved this book into what it is today. Thank you to Lynn Pentz, Dr. Michael Ryce, Dr. Rich Anderson, Irma Nippert, Shirley Bennett, Carolyn Dawson, Ruth Shelton, Michael Edwards, Sheridan Hill, and Andrea Hare.

To the many friends and family members who gave me lots of insightful feedback and encouragement along the way. Thank you to Don Tolman, Carolyn Dawson, Kavita Daswani, Neville Raymond, Irene Newman, Judith Johnson, Cheri Bowers, Ken Cadigan, Steve Tilton, Dino DeFilippi, Leonard Farrell, Joe Piscateli, Antanas Vainius, Sean Keenan, Gwendolyn Morton, Bill Bowers, Kathryn Phelps, Karen Ormstead, Chuck Peters, Summer Kolesar, James Taylor, Mary Anne Wise, Helene Abrams, David Giller, Sondra Ray and Mark Sullivan.

To Jodie Rhodes with Jodie Rhodes Literary Agency who believed that this manuscript should be "out there" and supported me in everyway possible.

To all my friends on the island of Patmos in Greece.

To Eija Storgard for creating such a magnificent book cover design.

To Sean Keenan for all of your encouragement and fabulous layout design.

To my sponsors whose financial contributions supported me greatly through the last few months of writing this book. Thank you to Rich Anderson and Arise & Shine, Carolyn Dawson, Gwendolyn and Philip Morton, Roxanne Bartels, and Paul Morton.

To Lorne Label, M.D., for taking the time while vacationing in Africa to read my manuscript and write the foreword to this book.

To Art Schwab, for being my most trusted friend throughout the years, and for believing in me and supporting me in every way.

INSIGHTS FROM THE AUTHOR

"Man did not weave the web of life…he is merely a strand in it.
Whatever he does to the web, he does to himself."

– Chief Seattle

The warning has been sounded. We're in the midst of an environmental crisis. Former U.S. vice-president Al Gore, now called "The Noah of our Times" by his colleagues, believes that global warming is threatening the very life of planet Earth. He has sounded an SOS signal, alerting us to the crisis at hand. In his book and documentary, *An Inconvenient Truth,* he declares that the burning of fossil fuel is the main culprit of global warming and if we will only "Answer the Call" and "Go Green," we can easily clean up the environment and turn our planet's environmental crisis around.

Other environmentalists disagree with Al Gore. They say that the burning of fossil fuel is *not* the main culprit of global warming and that the warming of our planet is occurring because of a much broader issue.

If this is true, the fact still remains: the burning of fossil fuel is polluting our planet. We are slowly but surely destroying our habitat. I know because some 25 years ago, I had almost destroyed mine. I woke up one morning and realized that not only had I been burning the wrong type of fuel in my car, but I had also been burning the wrong types of fuel in my body.

My body had sounded an SOS signal. I was in the midst of an internal environmental crisis. A type of global warming was threatening to take my life. I had a fever of 104 degrees that just wouldn't go away. Then one night, I collapsed from dehydration and was rushed to the hospital, where I was immediately admitted to an isolation room due to a dangerously low white blood cell count.

For days, my white blood cell count continued to drop, despite the many rounds of the strongest antibiotics possible. Even some of the most acclaimed allopathic experts had no clue as to the cause and therefore had no remedy for my potentially fatal condition. One physician simply blamed my declining white blood cell count on some mysterious germ and reported that if things didn't turn around, my life would soon come to an end.

But then, a new perspective was presented to me. Taylor, my friend and real estate broker, stopped by to see me and told me that he too had once been told that it might be too late for him. After doing extensive research as to why the human body becomes sick and dies, he began to shift his eating habits from an acidic meat-based, processed food diet to an alkaline plant-based, natural food diet. After a few short months, he experienced what others would call a miracle. Knowing that I, had been eating the SAD–Standard American Diet, laden with highly acidic, processed chemicalized foods, he encouraged me to do the same.

He looked up at my IV drip and told me that if I *truly* wanted to turn my crisis around, I needed to immediately check myself out of "man's" hospital and check myself into "nature's" hospital, where nature could heal me from the inside out. He told me that Hippocrates, the father of medicine, would turn over in his grave if he could see how the physicians of our time were using drugs as medicine instead of food.

> ### *"Let your food be your medicine and medicine be your food."*
> — Hippocrates,
> Father of Medicine

He went on to quote Hippocrates' famous statement, "Let your food be your medicine and medicine be your food."

He said that Hippocrates had based his entire healing practice on the observation and study of the human body as a whole and that a true physician was a teacher and the one who was sick was a student. To Hippocrates, the main duty of a physician is to simply standby and assist nature to strengthen the student's body, mind and spirit. He said that Hippocrates' goal was to *empower* his students by helping them understand that health is a natural effect of balance, and disease a result of imbalance.

To restore balance, Hippocrates trusted in nature to heal the body and the body to heal the mind. His prescribed medicines were whole foods, rest, enhanced elimination, cleanliness, fresh air and sunlight. He also used purges, enemas and fasting diets to evacuate toxicity from the body, the application of friction to increase circulation through massage, as well as the use of hot and cold water to further stimulate circulation.

As Taylor was leaving, he handed me some research papers that convinced me that he was right. I read how Antoine Béchamp, a 19th Century contemporary of Louis Pasteur, recognized that when the internal environment of the human body is in a state of balance, germs do not have a breeding ground. Since germs feed off of toxic waste, they simply cannot gain a foothold without a food supply. Pasteur and Béchamp each conducted prolific research into the cause of disease. They even worked side by side, but came to very different conclusions.

Pasteur believed that the interior of the human body is sterile and static like a spotlessly clean Petri dish. He believed that the cell is the elementary unit of life and hypothesized that harmful microbes were airborne and invaded the body, attacking us from the outside in, causing such physical reactions as fermentation, putrefaction and human disease. He taught that germs contaminate the tissue and cause disease, and that we are the prey, and the germs, the predators. This perspective is well known today as the *germ theory*.

Béchamp, on the other hand, believed that "disease is born of us and in us." He hypothesized that the cell couldn't be the elementary unit of life because there were certain microscopic entities within each cell that had the ability to evolve into bacteria under certain conditions and change their form. This pleomorphic activity takes place depending upon the environment the cells live in. He named these microscopic entities *microzymas*. He found that microzymas, based on the environment the cells live in, could not only change their form but their function as well, i.e. from helpful to hostile and back again, in countless variations. To his amazement, he found that microzymas were so strong that he was unable to destroy them at the highest of temperatures. He even found live microzymas in limestone dating to a geologic period some 60 million years ago when the first mammals appeared on Earth.

Béchamp discovered that microzymas are present in the tissues and blood of all living organisms where they remain benevolent and functional, especially in regards to cell division and immune function. He also discovered that when the welfare of the human body is threatened by the presence of potentially harmful material, such as accumulations of improperly digested foods and/or acids, a transmutation takes place. The microzymas change into a bacterium or virus, yeast or fungus, which immediately go to work to rid the body of this harmful material. Should the accumulated contamination continue to increase, the microorganisms would also continue to increase. What he discovered is that *when the environment is cleaned up,* the bacteria or viruses, yeast or fungus naturally reverted back to the microzyma's normal state of promoting life.

Thus, after much research, Béchamp concluded that the real cause of disease was *not* the germ, but rather an internal environment out of balance with nature and the natural order of things. Such imbalance is what makes the body a susceptible host to either external contamination or internal dissolution at the microscopic level. Or, as Béchamp is reputed to have said, "living beings, filled with microzymas, carry within themselves the elements essential for health or for disease, for life or for death."

> **When our internal environment is *clean* and *green,* disease cannot exist.**

Thus, his perspective was called the *internal terrain theory*, a theory that has never been refuted; one that reflects the internal message—the message that everything begins within us, and not the other way around.

Even though my family thought I had become insanely delirious from the high fever, Béchamp's internal terrain theory rang true to me, so I took my friend's advice and checked myself out of the hospital.

I was full of hope!

A few hours after my arrival at home, Taylor came by and delivered bags of organic food. He had everything from fruits and vegetables to nuts and seeds. It all seemed so strange to me. He had also brought me a high-powered juicer and blender, along with an assortment of self-help books on the healing power of food and periodic juice fasting as well as a book on how to clean out the accumulated toxic waste. I read all day and through the wee hours of the night.

Needless to say, my two children rebelled when I offered them carrot juice and whole grain cereal instead of a microwaved sticky bun for breakfast. But I was on a mission, not just to heal myself, but to make sure my family stayed healthy as well.

For the next 90 days, I went on a sabbatical. Work had taken a backseat. I read every book I could find on natural healing. Not only did I take Hippocrate's advice and heal myself with whole foods, fresh air, sunlight, water and a cleanse program that would evacuate the toxicity from my body, the totality of that experience caused insights to unfold within me which changed my life forever and prepared me for my destiny.

I became a student of nature and natural cures. Over the years, my desire for knowledge on how to achieve perfect health took me all over the world. I traveled extensively, visiting and studying at various holistic healing centers where I received several certifications in food and herbal nutrition. My studies revealed that modern day diseases increased as the contemporary American diet increased in net acid load relative to diets of the ancestral pre-agricultural *Homo sapiens.* This shift possibly occurred because of the agricultural revolution and the ubiquity of processed grains and shelf-stable food products high in chemicals and devoid of essential nutrients. Then fad diets became the norm; the latest trend being a diet high in animal protein foods and low in phytochemical plant foods from fresh fruits and vegetables.

Studies show that high protein diets derived from cheese, meat, fish and grains, increase net dietary acid load and acidify the urinary pH. Conversely, plant-based diets high in fruits and vegetables increase net dietary alkaline load and alkalize the urinary pH. Over time, ingestion of a high dietary acid load can progress into a chronic low-grade level of metabolic acidosis. This incidence of low-grade acidosis resulting from our modern diet has been well documented to cause a number of health conditions such as osteoporosis, cancer, heart disease, kidney disease, kidney stone formation, and muscle wasting. This chronic acid load creates an acid-alkaline imbalance, which in turn sets the conditions for germs to evolve to feed off the environment that acid waste creates.

After years of studies and bringing my own internal terrain back into a perfect state of balance, I discovered that the cause of my illness was, in fact, an overly acidic internal terrain produced from all the acidic foods I had been eating throughout the years; foods that were highly processed and full of chemicals, which provided a perfect feeding ground for the germ that had threatened to take my life. The germ was the effect of a toxic internal environment, which in turn had lowered my immunity. The germ was not the cause. In other words, *if you feed 'em, they'll come!*

What we have long called disease, and tag each one with a name, is simply a result of moving away from a perfect state of balance.

Disease means:
Dis **to move away from**
Ease **a perfect state of harmony**

Then, the cleaner and healthier my body became, the cleaner and healthier my mind became. This is when I began to view the world through the eyes of oneness. I could see that our earth's environmental crisis is a mere reflection of our body's environmental crisis. How we are polluting the earth is the same way we are polluting ourselves. Like burning the wrong type of fuel (fossil fuel) in our cars that adversely affects the outer environment, most of us are burning the wrong types of fuel (animal and processed foods loaded with chemicals) in our bodies that adversely affects our internal environment. This fuel not only creates a type of internal global warming, but an internal acid rain as well.

> *Burning the wrong types of food for fuel creates a type of internal acid rain.*

If you will, take a moment and ask yourself the same questions I had to ask myself: has the intelligence that runs your body been sending you an SOS signal? Have you been ignoring its distress call? Or have you been aware of it, attempting to listen, but unable to decipher the message? Could pain and disease be the SOS signal your body's intelligence is sending, attempting to warn you that you're burning the wrong types of food into the environment of your body, an alarm going off to get you to respond and "Answer the Call?"

I believe it is. The insights that are about to unfold in the following chapters are amazing. The basis of these insights has do with your body's ecology experiencing what I call an "ecological breakdown." However, what I discovered is that if you will heed your body's SOS signal, clean up your environment and change the types of food you're burning for fuel, your personal crisis would come to an end. The outer would follow simply; that is, you would begin to treat the earth as you treat yourself.

Thus, in order to affect real change and shift our planet's environmental crisis, we need to "be the change" and shift the crisis within ourselves by *getting clean* and *going green.*

So that's what I did, and that's why I'm still alive today, sounding my *Get Clean Go Green EcoDiet* message!

PART ONE

BE THE CHANGE!

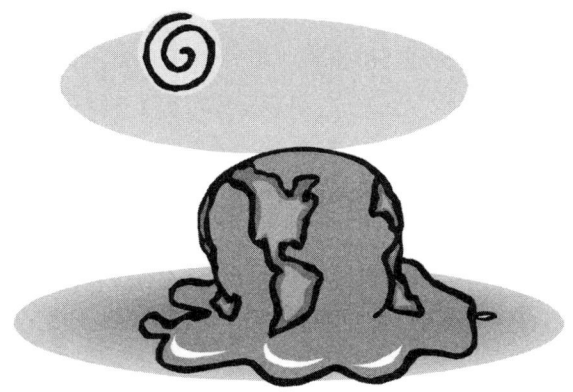

CHAPTER ONE

What is an EcoDiet?

When most of us hear the word "diet," we tend to think of a weight loss program; something we go on one day then off the next. Some may even think of it in the context of a health care professional telling us that we need to change to a healthier diet if our cholesterol or blood sugar is too high. But according to Merriam Webster, the word "diet" means "food and drink regularly provided or consumed." Another definition is "habitual nourishment." Thus, diet is a way of saying; something we consume on a regular basis, without ruthless caloric restrictions—just tossing out some bad stuff and adding some healthier choices to what most of us consume everyday.

So when we hear in the news that we should add something like olive oil to our diet, it just means that we should chuck the trans-fat laden hydrogenated gunk we're eating and substitute something that's healthier for our heart instead.

Since there's so much confusion around the word "diet," I chose the main title of my book, *EcoDiet,* after much deliberation.

The word "eco" means, environment or ecology; the word "diet" means, daily fare or a prescribed way of living. Mostly used as a prefix, "eco" is often added to an existing word to create another word with new meaning, mostly related to ecology. For example, eco-system, eco-house, eco-printing, etc., suggests a product that supports the environment or ecology of the earth.

Thus, an *EcoDiet* suggests an environmentally friendly way of eating—a daily fare that supports the ecology of our bodies, and a person who follows an *EcoDiet* is a *Body Ecologist,* a title I have given to myself.

A *Body Ecologist* is a person who studies the relationship between living things within their internal environment, and examines the effect of particular foods that support the ecological balance of their ecology. The basic principle they follow is that everything within their internal environment is connected and is designed to work together harmoniously, even though at the present time it may not be. Interested in their own personal environmental sustainability issues, they do everything possible to maintain ecological balance or to solve an already existing ecological imbalance by examining where they might have gone against nature and the natural order of things, such as the over consumption of foods that create an acid load, a lack of drinking enough purified water or taking in enough fresh air or sunlight.

In short, a *Body Ecologist* follows the principles an *EcoDiet* because they know that this recommended daily fare is the key to maintaining ecological health and a perfect state of balance. They understand that their body is a living ecosystem and because of this understanding, they become a devout student of their inner ecology and in turn teach others to do the same.

ECOSYSTEMS DEFINED

A living ecosystem is a natural unit consisting of a community of interdependent living organisms such as plants, animals, and microorganisms that live symbiotically in the environment they inhabit. The ecology of an ecosystem consists of the relationships and interactions between every living organism and its natural or unnatural environments. An ecosystem can consist of any form or any size—a log, pond, lake, field, forest, the earth's biosphere, and even the human body.

The main source of energy for every ecosystem is the sun. In fact, the health and wellbeing of every living organism begins and ends with the sun. Plants capture the sun's energy and use it to convert inorganic compounds into energy-rich organic compounds. This process of using the sun's energy to convert minerals such as magnesium or nitrogen from the soil into plant growth is called photosynthesis. The sun's energy is transformed and then made available to other living organisms through a pathway known as the food chain. In the hierarchy of the food chain, each group feeds on the group below it.

This way of feeding can be used to divide every living creature existing within the same ecosystem into three categories: producer organisms, consumer organisms and reducer organisms.

Green plants are producer organisms

Through the process of photosynthesis, green plants produce the food upon which all other organic life depends. They are called producer organisms because they convert solar energy directly into complex compounds that either form the body of the plant itself or are stored as seeds, nuts and fruits. Green plants form the entire beginning of the food chain. *Rich in chlorophyll, green plants are amongst the most alkalizing foods available.*

Herbivores are consumer organisms

Animals such as deer, rabbits, cattle, pigs, squirrels, and seed-eating birds are called consumer organisms because they acquire their energy second-hand from consuming green plants or their nuts, seeds and fruits. *Like primates, scientific evidence suggests that humans are also herbivores by ecological design as described in Chapter Two.*

Omnivores are secondary consumer organisms

Omnivores such as opossums, pigs, bears, chickens, emus and a variety of birds eat both plant foods and meat for their sustenance and are therefore mixed primary and secondary consumer organisms.

Carnivores are secondary consumer organisms

Carnivores such as owls, vultures, wolves, and bobcats are called secondary consumer organisms because they derive their energy from eating the herbivores.

Microorganisms are reducer organisms

Microbes such as bacteria, fungi, yeast, parasites, and algae are called reducer organisms because their inherent function is to decompose and devour all that is dead and dying back into the dust of the earth, thus cleaning up the environment for the living. Often perceived as germs or pests, reducer organisms are a misunderstood and necessary part of the food chain.

If any environment provides reducer organisms
with a food supply, rest assured…they will come!

In the following chapters, we'll explore dietary devolution, the human body and how I believe it, like the ecology of the earth, loses its natural state of balance, and becomes diseased to the point of death. Just know that I believe, no matter what your condition or what disease name you may have been tagged with, it's never too late to turn your environmental crisis around.

I did, and so can you!

CHAPTER TWO

Dietary Devolution

We have clearly moved far away from a plant-based alkaline diet that supports our natural ecological design. The devolution began when we shifted from an herbivore diet to an omnivore diet, one of eating both plants and animals. We then shifted from an omnivore diet to a chemivore diet to a junkitarian diet. The entire scope of dietary devolution is not only harmful to our inner ecology, but to the ecology of the earth itself. Dietary devolution can be characterized by these three distinct measures: (1) the ingesting of animal foods and their byproducts, (2) foods that contain chemical residue from living in toxic waters, toxic habitats or being grown on toxic fields and (3) foods that have been processed and are loaded with toxic chemicals. These three categories of food are extremely acid-forming to the human body and, when acid rains, it destroys everything it touches.

DIETARY DEVOLUTION #1
From Herbivore to Omnivore

Scientific observation, along with good old-fashioned common sense, suggests that humans, by "eco"-logical and "bio"-logical design, are herbivores, not omnivores, as some would suggest. This means that we are primary consumer organisms, created to acquire our nourishment from green plants, nuts, seeds, and fruits.

Cardiologist William C. Roberts, M.D., hails from the famed cattle state of Texas. He unequivocally believes that humans aren't physiologically designed to eat meat; that when we kill animals to eat them, they end up killing us because their flesh, which contains cholesterol and saturated fat, was never intended for human beings.

Another consideration is that 80% of breast, bowel and prostate cancers are attributed to dietary practices, and international comparisons show strong positive associations with meat consumption. Dr. Roberts said, "I think the evidence is pretty clear. If you look at various characteristics of carnivores versus herbivores, it doesn't take a genius to see where humans line up."

Milton R. Mills, M.D., associate director of preventive medicine for the Physicians Committee for Responsible Medicine (PCRM) reports in his study, "The Comparative Anatomy of Eating," that we simply aren't physiologically designed to eat meat, even though we have been conditioned to do so through cultural habituation. While most humans are clearly behavioral omnivores, the question to answer is whether humans are anatomically suited for a diet that includes animal as well as plant foods. To answer this question, we need to make a comparative examination of the typical anatomy and physiology of carnivores, omnivores and herbivores in the animal world and compare their attributes with those of the human body.

Biologists have established that animals that share physical characteristics also share a common diet.

COMPARATIVE ANATOMY OF EATING CHART

FEATURE	CARNIVORE	HERBIVORE	OMNIVORE	HUMAN
FACIAL MUSCLES	Reduced to allow wide mouth gape	Well-developed	Reduced	Well-developed
JAW TYPE	Angle not expanded	Expanded angle	Angle not expanded	Expanded angle
JAW JOINT LOCATION	On same plane as molar teeth	Above the plane of the molars	On same plane as molar teeth	Above the plane of the molars
JAW MOTION	Shearing; minimal side-to-side motion	No shear; good side-to-side, front-to-back	Shearing; minimal side-to-side	No shear; good side-to-side, front-to-back
MAJOR JAW MUSCLES	Temporalis	Masseter and pterygoids	Temporalis	Masseter and pterygoids
MOUTH OPENING vs. HEAD SIZE	Large	Small	Large	Small

TEETH: INCISORS	Short and pointed	Broad, flattened and spade shaped	Short and pointed	Broad, flattened and spade shaped
TEETH: CANINES	Long, sharp and curved	Dull and short or long (for defense), or none	Long, sharp and curved	Short and blunted
TEETH: MOLARS	Sharp, jagged and blade shaped	Flattened with cusps vs. complex surface	Sharp blades and/or flattened	Flattened with nodular cusps
CHEWING	None; swallows food whole	Extensive chewing necessary	Swallows food whole and/or simple crushing	Extensive chewing necessary
SALIVA	No digestive enzymes	Carbohydrate digesting enzymes	No digestive enzymes	Carbohydrate digesting enzymes
STOMACH TYPE	Simple	Simple or multiple chambers	Simple	Simple
STOMACH ACIDITY	Less than or equal to pH 1 with food in stomach	pH 4 to 5 with food in stomach	Less than or equal to pH 1 with food in stomach	pH 4 to 5 with food in stomach
STOMACH CAPACITY	60% to 70% of total volume of digestive tract	Less than 30% of total volume of digestive tract	60% to 70% of total volume of digestive tract	21% to 27% of total volume of digestive tract
LENGTH OF SMALL INTESTINE	3 to 6 times body length	10 to more than 12 times body length	4 to 6 times body length	10 to 11 times body length
COLON	Simple, short and smooth, no fermentation	Long, complex; may be sacculated, may ferment	Simple, short and smooth, no fermentation	Long, sacculated, may ferment
LIVER	Can detoxify vitamin A	Cannot detoxify vitamin A	Can detoxify vitamin A	Cannot detoxify vitamin A
KIDNEY	Extremely concentrated urine	Moderately concentrated urine	Extremely concentrated urine	Moderately concentrated urine
NAILS	Sharp claws	Flattened nails or blunt hooves	Sharp claws	Flattened nails
THERMOSTASIS	Hyperventilation	Perspiration	Hyperventilation	Perspiration

Adapted from the article *"The Comparative Anatomy of Eating"*
by Milton R. Mills, M.D.

In 2001, a group of endocrinologists at the University of California-San Francisco were wondering whether acid animal protein sources would have different effects than a diet relatively higher in alkaline plant proteins. In fact, in a study of over 1,000 elderly women, they found that a higher reliance on animal sources of protein significantly increased bone loss and the chances of hip fractures. The next year, they followed up this study with an analysis of changes in the human diet, from the hunter-gatherer societies of the past to the contemporary diet of industrialized nations. What they found was astounding. A huge transformation has taken place in the human internal metabolic environment.

Until recently, human beings lived with continuous, but mild, systemic alkalosis, the result of a predominantly plant-based alkaline diet, and relative, by today's standards, disease free. Today, due to the devolution of our diet, human beings are mostly living in a mild to severe state of acidosis, which may be the link to the exponential increase of disease during the last 60 years.

Study after study has shown links between meat and dairy consumption and chronic diseases that send millions of people to the grave each year. Epidemiological results reported in the book, *The China Study*, published in 2005, documents these facts.

This study documents the results of the 20-year research project directed by medical researcher T. Colin Campbell, Ph.D., and his son, Thomas M. Campbell II, in a partnership between Cornell University, Oxford University, and the Chinese Academy of Preventive Medicine. They compare the results of that study with a number of other provocative studies, thus *The New York Times* called it the "most comprehensive large study ever undertaken of the relationship between diet and the risk of developing disease."

The *China Study* produced more than 8,000 statistically significant associations between various dietary factors and disease. The main conclusion of this study revealed that people who primarily ate animal-based foods developed more chronic diseases, while people who primarily ate plant-based foods were healthier. They found abundant evidence linking diets high in protein, particularly animal protein (including casein in cow's milk), to chronic degenerative diseases. They go so far as to say, "even relatively small intakes of animal-based foods were *associated with adverse effects.*"

An article entitled, *Red-meat Diet Ups Odds of Early Death,* by Rob Stein of the Washington Post, published March 24, 2009, summarized a study led by Rashmi Sinha of the National Cancer Institute, which was published in the Archives of Internal Medicine. It revealed the following:

- Eating red meat increases the chances of dying prematurely, according to a large federal study that offers powerful new evidence that a diet that regularly includes steaks, burgers and pork chops is hazardous to your health.

- The study of more than 500,000 middle-aged and elderly Americans found that those who consumed the equivalent of about a small hamburger every day were more than 30% more likely to die during the ten years they were followed, mostly from heart disease and cancer. Sausage, cold cuts and other processed meats also increased the risk.

- Previous research had found a link between red meat and an increased risk of heart disease and cancer, particularly colorectal cancer, but the new study is the first large examination of the relationship between eating meat and overall mortality.

- Women who ate the most red meat were 36% more likely to die for any reason, 20% more likely to die from cancer and 50% more likely to die from heart disease. Men who ate the most meat were 31% more likely to die for any reason, 22% more likely to die of cancer and 27% more likely to die of heart disease.

Another major factor to consider about the shift from an herbivore diet to an omnivore diet is the devastation of our planet.

A 2006 United Nations report summarized the devastation caused by the meat industry by calling it "one of the top two or three most significant contributors to the most serious environmental problems, at every scale from local to global." The report recommended that animal agriculture "be a major policy focus when dealing with problems of land degradation, climate change and air pollution, water shortage and water pollution, and loss of biodiversity."

Many leading environmental organizations, such as the National Audubon Society and the Sierra Club, are now establishing the link between eating meat and eco-disasters like climate change. According to Environmental Defense, if every American skipped one meal of chicken per week and substituted vegetarian foods instead, the carbon dioxide savings would be the same as taking more than a half-million cars off U.S. roads.

Eating 1 lb. of meat emits the same amount of greenhouse gasses as driving an SUV 40 miles.

Environmental impacts of eating animals include:

Wasted Resources	Pollution
Land	Feces
Food	Water
Energy	Air
Water	Global Warming
Rainforest	
Animal Suffering	

DIETARY DEVOLUTION #2
From Herbivore to Omnivore to Chemivore

In recent years, the issue of eating at the top of the food chain has taken an even more disturbing turn. Arctic waters, while relatively pristine with contamination levels of 10 to 100 times lower than the Great Lakes, are becoming toxic; chemicals from the fall-out of agriculture, jet exhaust, and industrial manufacturing plants, along with the burning of fossil fuel, have reached to the farthest corners of the earth, carried by rivers, ocean currents, and winds. Aquatic life in the Arctic feed from the water's plankton, and plankton derives its nutrients from the ocean's waters. But in the process of collecting nutrients, (a process called bioaccumulation), toxic pollutants are also accumulated, making them much more concentrated in the cells of the plankton than in the open water.

Because small fish eat vast amounts of plankton, these toxic chemicals collect and concentrate in their flesh. This process is called bio-magnification and is repeated at each step of the food chain. Predators four to five links up on the food chain are found to have accumulations of toxic chemicals in their tissues millions of times higher than that of the water they inhabit. Thus, scientists are finding hundreds of hazardous synthetic compounds in the flesh of those who inhabit the Arctic tundra, at levels so extreme that the breast milk and tissues of some Greenlander people could be classified as hazardous waste.

While this example might be considered a worst-case scenario of why we should reconsider eating our foods from the top of the food chain, it isn't.

Large fish such as shark, king mackerel, swordfish, and tuna eat various types of food in the contaminated mercury-ridden waters they swim in. Golden bass and snapper have much higher amounts of mercury than any other type of fish. Although more in-depth studies are needed to determine how much mercury it takes to negatively affect us, the bottom line is that enough studies are out to prove that it in fact does.

Some studies report that even low levels of mercury can be extremely toxic. Babies who were exposed to even tiny doses of mercury before birth can have slower reflexes, speech problems, and even autism. Infants contaminated by mercury can even have a broad range of disabilities including blindness, deafness, cerebral palsy and mental retardation amongst others. The USDA warns children and women who are pregnant or women who might become pregnant, to avoid eating seafood. Even so, consumer demands for seafood have increased in the U.S.

To support growing consumer demand, opportunities emerged for aqua-culturalists to profit from producing farm-raised fish grown on farms or in other managed environments. Farm-raised fish factories have doubled over the past decade and are now "one of the fastest growing food producing sectors," according to the United Nations' Food and Agriculture Organization (FAO). Today, approximately one in five fish consumed worldwide is raised in captivity.

From the temperature-controlled hatching tanks, small growing fish are transferred to the small rearing areas where they grow to maturity, having little or no room to swim or breathe. Raising fish in crowded, excrement-laden water necessitates the broad use of agrichemicals. An FDA veterinarian article explains that fish farmers "use chemicals as disinfectants and to kill bacteria; herbicides to prevent the overgrowth of vegetation in ponds; vaccines to fight certain diseases; and drugs, usually combined in the feed, to treat diseases and parasites." As a result, the potential exists for consumers of farm-raised fish to ingest residues of these drugs and chemicals. The ingestion of these drugs and chemicals can and do produce long-term health concerns.

In 2002, the U.S. Geological Survey (USGS) released the first study of pharmaceuticals, hormones, and other organic chemicals in waterways across the nation. Ninety-five chemicals were measured and detected at very low concentrations; there were no drinking-water standards for 81 of these. Antibiotics, steroids, insect repellents, natural and synthetic hormones, plasticizers, and other human and veterinary drugs were among those tested and found. These chemicals come from the waters released from sewage treatment plants and from urban and agricultural runoff, and eventually appear again in our drinking water.

Factory-Farmed Animals

Animals raised for massive food consumption are unfortunately handled as units of production rather than living, breathing creatures. This mechanized approach ignores animals' inherent needs, which often sacrifices their health and wellbeing in the name of production as well as higher profits. Although there is controversy surrounding the degrees of comfort and freedom that farm animals should have, most people agree that farm animals deserve a minimum standard of cleanliness and space and don't need to suffer needlessly.

Confining animals indoors, as closely together as possible, rather than letting them roam and graze on open pastures, exposes the animals to high levels of toxins, which are released when so much manure decomposes in an enclosed space. To counteract the disease inherent in such conditions, animals are given constant doses of antibiotics.

Not only are animals fed constant doses of drugs to counterbalance disease conditions, they are also fed various drugs in an effort to maximize their growth and market value in the shortest time possible. It has been discovered that meat slaughtered from animals raised in factory farms contain drugs such as growth hormones, steroids as well as antibiotic residues. It is estimated that animals that receive antibiotics in their feed often gain 4-5% more body weight than animals that do not receive the drug. Sadly, more than 24.6 million pounds of antibiotics are added to livestock feed every year. This adds up to about half of the amount manufactured in the United States.

A report from the National Research Council has acknowledged that there is a link between the use of antibiotics in food animals, the development of bacterial resistance to these drugs, and human disease. Antibiotic-resistant bacteria inevitably develop in cattle, and can easily be transmitted to humans through the consumption of meat or through human contact with living animals. This leads to a reduction in the efficiency of antibiotics in fighting infections, reduced levels of favorable intestinal bacteria, which increases susceptibility to intestinal infections, such as acute gastroenteritis with fever, pain and diarrhea. A depressed immune system also results, which could lower resistance to infections and increase allergic reactions. Those at the greatest risk include infants, the elderly and those with weakened immune systems.

And, unfortunately, it doesn't stop with our livestock. The pig, poultry, dairy and egg industries employ technological short cuts such as drugs, hormones, and other chemicals to maximize production. These animals experience cruelty beyond belief, from birth to slaughter, just to feed our growing demands. Under these inhumane conditions, virulent pathogens are emerging that are resistant to antibiotics. These new superbugs, whose evolution is traceable directly to the overuse of antibiotics, have the potential to cause massive human suffering.

Mad Cow Disease (Bovine spongiform encephalopathy-BSE), a fatal neurode-generative disease-affecting cattle that spread throughout Britain in 1996 when dead cows were fed to living cows, is a rude example of factory-farmed animals. This insidious disease causes a spongy degeneration in the brain and spinal cord. In the United Kingdom, the country worst affected, more than 179,000 cattle have been infected and 4.4 million slaughtered during the eradication program. When people ate these "cannibalistic" diseased cows, they contracted Creutzfeldt-Jakob Disease (CJD), a fatal dementia that affects humans.

By February 2009, it had killed 164 people in Britain and 42 elsewhere with the number expected to rise because of the disease's long incubation period. Between 460,000 and 482,000 BSE-infected animals had entered the food chain before controls on high-risk offal (edible internal organs) were introduced in 1989. A British inquiry into BSE concluded that the epidemic was caused by cattle, which are normally herbivores, being fed the remains of other cattle in the form of meat and bone meal, which caused the infectious agent to spread.

Another factory-farm tragedy that jeopardizes both animals and humans is avian influenza, an infection caused by avian (bird) influenza (flu) viruses. Another name for avian influenza is bird flu. In Hong Kong, where scores of people have died from the so-called bird flu, over one million chickens have been destroyed in the panic to stop the spread of the disease. Symptoms of avian influenza in humans have ranged from typical human influenza-like symptoms, such as fever, cough, sore throat, and muscle aches to eye infections, pneumonia, severe respiratory diseases, and other severe and life-threatening complications. The avian influenza virus that has crossed the species barrier to infect humans, H5N1, has caused the largest number of detected cases of severe disease and death in humans.

The reported conclusion is that millions of people around the world are infected and thousands die every year from consuming contaminated animal food products. Rather than advising consumers to curtail their intake of animal foods, the agribusiness industry devised extreme measures, such as overcooking and antibiotics, to help consumers circumvent the hazards of eating these sick and diseased animals.

And while these are only a few examples, the effect of factory farming is immense and widespread, all of which includes the despoliation of the earth.

According to research conducted by John Robbins, founder of Earth Save Foundation, methane gas (from animal farts!) is responsible for nearly as much global warming as all other non-CO_2 greenhouse gases put together. Methane, being 21 times more powerful a greenhouse gas than CO_2, causes nearly half of the planet's human-induced warming. Therefore, methane reduction must be a priority. The number one source of methane worldwide is animal agriculture, which produces more than 100 million tons of methane per year. About 85% of methane gas is produced in the digestive processes of livestock and, while a single cow releases a relatively small amount of methane, the collective effect on the environment of hundreds of millions of livestock animals worldwide is enormous.

Environmental impacts of factory-farming can also include:

• Deforestation for animal feed production.

- Unsustainable pressure on the land for the production of high- protein/high energy animal feed.

- Deforestation for animal feed production.

- Pesticide, herbicide and fertilizer manufacture and use for feed production.

- Unsustainable use of water for feed-crops, including groundwater   extraction.

- Pollution of soil, water and air by nitrogen and phosphorous from fertilizer used for feed-crops and from manure.

- Land degradation (reduced fertility, soil compaction, increased salinity, desertification).

- Loss of biodiversity due to eutrophication, acidification, pesticides and herbicides.

- Worldwide reduction of genetic diversity of livestock and loss of traditional breeds.

- Species extinctions due to livestock-related habitat destruction (especially feed-cropping).

In essence, a global solution for both our inner our outer environmental crisis could be as simple as this; that is, to completely eliminate the consumption of animals and animal products and become the herbivores we were created to be.

Chemical Agriculture

The ever-increasing pollution of the environment has been one of the greatest concerns for both science and the general public for the last 50 years. With the rapid industrialization of agriculture, the need for food transportation, the ever-expansion of the chemical industry, and the irrationality of genetically modified seeds, the atmosphere, bodies of water, and many soil environments have become polluted by a huge variety of toxic compounds. Many of these compounds used at high concentrations or following prolonged exposure have the potential to produce adverse effects for humans as well as other organisms. These include the danger of acute tissue toxicity, genetic changes, carcinogenesis, and birth defects. Some of these man-made toxic compounds are also resistant to physical, chemical, or biological degradation and thus represent an environmental burden of considerable magnitude.

Consequently, our agricultural food supply gravely suffers.

- It contains pesticide residue.

- It is irradiated.

- It is shipped great distances.

- It is chemical intensive.

- It may be genetically engineered.

- (GMO—genetically modified organisms)

In the early 1900s, the majority of people living in the U.S. were farmers who produced food for themselves as well as others living in surrounding communities. Today, less than 2% of the U.S. populations are considered farmers. Large agribusiness corporations whose interests are in maximizing profits are growing our food. As a result, large amounts of petrochemicals, artificial fertilizers, and toxic pesticides are used. The attempt is then made to increase soil fertility and reduce destruction to crops from pests by spending billions of dollars and applying billions of pounds of chemicals to the land and food. The result is the destruction of the microbial life of the soil and an imbalance of beneficial insects.

In 1987, the Environmental Protection Agency (EPA) stated that pesticide residue in food is one of the nation's three most serious health hazards. Various toxic pesticides that have been outlawed and banned in the U.S. are often used on crops in many foreign countries whose food growing requirements are less stringent than ours. The insane thing is that we then import the produce from these countries, which makes us again vulnerable to ingesting the chemical residues. Sadly, only a small percentage of the billions of pounds of food imported into the U.S. today are inspected for specific pesticide residues. Some pesticides are not tested for at all, making it likely that we are ingesting a greater amount of pesticide residue than what is considered safe and reasonable by the FDA.

Approximately one-half of the amount of pesticides used are to make produce appealing to the eye. A variety of unhealthy waxes that contain other chemicals such as fungicides are used to coat our produce to help with shelf life and transportation.

These waxes and fungicide residues are very difficult to wash off of fruits and vegetables, and peeling the skin does not always help either, as they are often absorbed into the flesh of the produce.

Pesticide, herbicide and fungicide residue in our food increases the chance for serious illness and disease in adults as well as children. Children are at a much higher risk to pesticide exposure due to the fact that they ingest a greater amount of food per pound of body weight. By age five, millions of children have ingested up to 35% of an entire lifetime dose of some carcinogenic pesticides. From 1973 to 1990, nervous system and brain cancers rose 32% in children and leukemia was up 27% in children.

According to Robert Buist, Ph.D., in his book, *Food Chemical Sensitivity,* given the typical modern diet, together with the constant increase in new synthetic chemicals, an estimated 50,000 different chemicals enter our body from the following sources: food additives, pesticides, herbicides, drugs, and household and industrial chemicals.

Only a small percentage of the billions of pounds of food imported into the U.S. today are inspected for specific pesticide residues.

These toxic, acidic chemicals are now in the air you breathe, the water you drink, the oceans you swim in, the food you eat, and the personal care and household products you use. Dr. Buist informed us approximately 22 years ago that our body's elimination systems were simply overwhelmed and unable to keep up with this overload of toxic chemicals. At that time the average American was already consuming more than five pounds of chemical ingredients every year.

Paula Baillie-Hamilton, M.D., author of *The Body Restoration Plan* warns of the pervasive nature of pesticides and other synthetic chemicals, which are mostly created from petroleum. She noted the ever-increasing role of petroleum as a basis of our society through the last century parallels the every increasing role of acidosis as a basis of the diseases from which we suffer in the industrialized world. She writes that the same common classes of pesticides that are found in trace amounts in commercially grown foods (organophosphates, organochlorines, and carbamates) have historically been added in very low doses to feed to fatten livestock. These pesticides, along with residual doses of steroids and antibiotics, reduce the metabolic rate, making less feed go further, and reduce the ability to burn existing fat stores. In addition, they break down the structure of muscle fibers, reduce the ability to produce energy to power exercise, essentially reduce the desire to move, and accelerate weight gain.

These are only a few impacts that chemical agriculture has on our environment:

- In the United States alone, approximately 40 percent of all chemical fertilizers used eventually break down into ammonia and are released into the atmosphere.

- Researchers from the Department of Economics at the University of Essex put the annual cost of environmental damage caused by industrial farming in the United States at $34.7 billion.

- An important national issue is the degradation of water quality from nonpoint sources of pollution, including the prevalent use of fertilizers and pesticides on agricultural land. Nutrients from fertilizers encourages the growth of algae, which leads to low oxygen levels in streams and the possibility of fish kills.

- The excessive use of fertilizers, herbicides, fungicides and pesticides on a regular basis causes extensive environmental hazards because the majority of these toxic chemicals either do not undergo biodegradation or they undergo degradation (by microorganisms or ultraviolet light) releasing pollutants in the environment.

Thus, a global solution for both our inner our outer environmental crisis could be as simple as this; that is, to return to a more organic, biodiverse way of farming.

Food Irradiation

One of the latest additions to the long line of food devolution is the exposure of our food to radioactivity with the intent to extend its shelf life. Foods being irradiated include meats, grains, herbs, and produce. To date, there is no government food requirement to label food that has been irradiated. Commercially grown food is generally bombarded with radiation 5,000 to 1,000,000 times greater than a chest x-ray. The results of this exposure are two-fold, (1) the destruction of vital nutrients and vitamins, and an alteration of the chemical structure of the food and (2) the health risk and long term effects of chemical compounds developed in the food as a result of radioactive exposure.

Genetically Modified Food

Genetically modified organisms (GMO) are life forms that have been genetically engineered. Genetic engineering is a laboratory technique used by scientists to change the DNA (the blueprint for the individuality of an organism) of living organisms. This is a process of taking genes from one strain of a plant, animal or virus, and inserting them into another with the goal of reproducing chosen characteristics of the original species in the receiving species. Genetic engineering uses materials from organisms that have never been a part of the human food supply to change the fundamental nature of the food we eat. Without long-term testing, no one knows if these foods are safe. These scientists are experimenting with very delicate, yet powerful forces of nature without full knowledge of widespread repercussions. As with pesticides and drugs, safety testing for GMOs is not performed by the companies that produce them, raising public concern about financial motives and gain, ethics and conflict of interest. Europe and India are amongst two countries that are trying to ban GMO seeds.

DIETARY DEVOLUTION #3
From Herbivore to Omnivore to Chemivore to Junkivore

According to the USDA's Economic Research Service (ERS) food expenditure statistics for 2005, Americans spend an average of 9.9% of their disposable income on food. Regrettably, 90% of those dollars are spent on processed foods loaded with toxic chemicals. These nutrient-deprived foods are at the bottom of the devolution food chain and contain:

- Artificial colors.
- Artificial flavors.
- Artificial sweeteners.

- Preservatives.
- Highly processed salt, oil and sugar.
- Numerous other man-made ingredients to help in the manufacturing, appearance, texture, flavor, color, and shelf life of the product.

For profit and growing public demand, food processing companies are manufacturing and packaging everything from frozen and canned foods, macaroni and cheese, TV dinners, burgers and fries, luncheon meats and white bread, jellies and jams, noodles and sauce, mayonnaise and ketchup, hot dogs and bologna, crackers and cheese, instant mashed potatoes and gravy, powdered eggs and pasteurized milk, instant and boxed cereals, and the list goes on. In addition, processed food manufacturers load their products with the cheapest materials possible. These substances include hydrogenated oils, refined salt and sugar (such as sucrose, glucose, dextrose, and high fructose corn syrup), artificial sweeteners and colors (such as sodium benzoate, sulfites, nitrates, nitrites, BHT and MSG)—all to brighten the color, enhance flavor and ensure a long shelf life.

As an example, the secret ingredient in a famous fried chicken recipe is MSG (monosodium glutamate), a flavor-enhancing chemical compound, which provides a savory taste to food. In 1959, the FDA classified MSG as a "generally recognized as safe" food additive under the Federal Food, Drug and Cosmetic Act, and is now a widely used additive in the food industry. While the U.S. government currently has no restrictions or warnings on MSG, numerous scientists from around the world have repeatedly confirmed that MSG in the diet causes a range of health problems in animals, including obesity. In 2008, researchers at the University of North Carolina at Chapel Hill, working with Chinese researchers, published a study that found a positive link between MSG intake and obesity in humans: the prevalence of being overweight was significantly higher in MSG users than in non-users. The population in this study was 752 healthy rural Chinese villagers between the ages of 40 and 59, of whom 48.7% were women.

The prevalence of being overweight is significantly higher in MSG users than in non-users.

Another example is aspartame, which is a synthetic sweetener used in most diet drinks. Aspartame is a protein produced from aspartic acid, an amino acid occurring in many plant proteins that can also be produced by humans and animals. When the temperature of Aspartame exceeds 86°F, the wood alcohol converts to formaldehyde and then to formic acid, which in turn causes metabolic acidosis. Aspartame is known to change the brain's chemistry, causing everything from severe seizures, neurological diseases, birth defects, memory loss, vertigo, depression, phobias, ADD, anxiety attacks, blindness, decreased vision, high blood pressure, fibromyalgia, lymphoma, and many other known and unknown disorders.

Janet Starr Hull, creator of the *Aspartame Detox Program*, calls aspartame "sweet poison." She states, "the dangers of aspartame poisoning have been a well-guarded secret since the 1980s. The research and history of aspartame is conclusive as a cause of illness and toxic reactions in the human body. Side effects can occur gradually, can be immediate, or can be acute reactions. It is a dangerous chemical food additive and its use during pregnancy and by children is one of the greatest modern tragedies of all."

According to Lendon Smith, M.D., an enormous segment of the population suffers from side effects associated with aspartame, yet most have no idea why drugs, supplements and herbs don't relieve their symptoms. There are users who don't appear to suffer immediate reactions at all. But even these individuals are susceptible to the long-term damage caused by excitatory amino acids, phenylalanine, methanol, and diketopiperazine (DKP).

Consumer beware! Did you know that? ...

- The commercial food industries add over 1,000 new chemicals into our food supply each and every year.

- The average American consumes over five pounds of chemicals each year that come from our food supply.

- As outlined in *Food Label News*, the FDA does not restrict the term "natural" on food labels provided the product is free of artificial flavors, chemical preservatives, or added colors.

My motto: if you can't read it, don't eat it!

Our food supply devolved even further down the toxic acidifying food chain with the production of empty-calorie junk foods, such as potato chips, corn chips, cola, candy, cookies, ice cream, cake, etc. These items are not only processed, they are loaded with highly refined products such as salt, oil, and sugar and most are loaded with chemicals that the general population can't even pronounce. These junk foods are amongst the most acidifying of them all.

Take a look at a list of the toxic chemicals included in the strawberry flavoring of a milkshake served at a fast-food drive-thru window.

> Amyl acetate, amyl butyrate, amyl valerate, anethol, anisyl formate, benzyl acetate, benzyl isobutyrate, butyric acid, cinnamyl isobutyrate, cinnamylvalerate, cognac essential oil, diacetyl, dipropyl ketone, ethyl butyrate, ethyl cinnamate, ethyl heptanoate, ethyl lactate, ethyl methylphenylglycidate, ethyl Nitrate, ethyl propionate, ethyl valerbate, heliotropin, hydroxphrenyl-2butanone (10% solution to alcohol), a-ionone, isobutyl anthranilate, isobutyl butrate, lemon essential oil, maltol, 4-methylacetophenone, methyl anthranilate, methyl benzoate, methyl cinnamate, methyl heptine carbone, methyl naphthyl ketone, methyl slicylate, mint essential oil, neroli essential oil, nerolin, neryl isobulyrate, orris butter, phenethyl alcohol, sore rum ether, g-undecalctone, vanillin, and solvent 3.

The meaning of a true vegetarian: Someone who eats vegetation!

Sadly, even some vegetarians have fallen into an acid-based junkitarian diet, as suggested by the *Urban Dictionary*. They define a junkitarian as someone who is technically a vegetarian in that they abstain from meat, but who negates all the potential health benefits by eating mostly junk food. Many teenagers have fallen into this category. It makes being a "vegetarian" really easy, since you still get to eat junk all the time, and still get the cool hippie status that comes with vegetarianism. However, a true vegetarian is defined as *someone who eats vegetation*…not someone who eats a diet high in processed foods, even if that food carries an organic, health food store label.

So before you take your next bite, ask yourself two things: (1) is the food I'm about to eat going to support the ecological health of my inner as well as my outer environment and (2) is this food I'm about to eat really food…or is it merely a potpourri of empty-calories and chemicals masking itself as food!?

CHAPTER THREE

The Power of pH

We live on a planet with limited resources with only one contribution from the atmosphere outside of us—the energy from the sun. The sun is the source that fuels life on our planet, working in harmony with the other elements to create for us an abundant existence. And even though modern day technologies and industries have the ability to use large bodies of water to generate electricity and to drill deep into the Earth to extract energy, the limits to this process have become evident. Not only that, but we use this energy to the detriment of our environment.

Not only are we out of harmony with our natural resources through windows of "narrow thinking," we are polluting our earth, our bodies, ourselves. A return to "ecological thinking" for ourselves as well as our planet is necessary if we are to survive.

Throughout this chapter, my hope is take you to another level of realization; that life on earth is held within ecosystems and ecosystems are based on balance. Balance is the key.

Now let's take a look into the anatomical make-up of the human body; how our body's ecology thrives and how, like the ecology of the earth, it becomes sick and dies.

THE HUMAN BODY & pH

Based on the chemical elements of the periodic table, the human body is, by weight, composed of 65% oxygen, 18% carbon, 10% hydrogen, 3% nitrogen along with various electrolyte minerals and trace mineral compounds. Soon, you will come to realize that, like the earth, our bodies are mostly made up of air, fire, earth, and water and, if we are out of harmony with these elemental forces of nature, we will eventually suffer the effects of an environmental crisis.

The following chart decodes the elemental composition of our physical existence.

The Human Body

Element	% Of Body Weight	Primary Systems Requiring This Element
Oxygen	65%	Bones, Teeth, Skin, Blood, Corpuscles, Circulation
Carbon	18%	Teeth, Skin, Connective Tissue, Hair, Nails
Hydrogen	10%	Blood and Cells
Nitrogen	3%	Muscles, Cartilage, Tissues, Ligaments, Tendons, Flesh
Calcium	2%	Bones and Teeth
Phosphorus	1%	Blood and Brain
Potassium	0.4%	Blood, Bones and Cells
Sulfur	0.25%	Blood
Sodium	0.25%	Skin, Nerves, Mucus Membranes
Chlorine	0.25%	Epithelium, Nerves
Fluorine	0.2%	Nails, Hair, Blood, Skin
Magnesium	0.05%	Blood, Nerves, Muscles
Iron	0.008%	Blood, Bones, Brain, Muscle
Manganese	0.003%	Hemoglobin, Lymph
Silicon	0.00002%	Blood, Muscles, Nerves, Skin, Nails, Hair
Iodine	0.00004%	Thyroid, Blood, Spinal Nerves, Brain, Bones Metabolism

Other known essential minerals that make up the human body include: zinc, silicon, rubidium, strontium, bromine, lead, copper, aluminum, cadmium, cerium, barium, iodine, tin, titanium, boron, nickel, selenium, chromium, manganese, arsenic, lithium, cesium, mercury, germanium, molybdenum, cobalt, antimony, silver, niobium, zirconium, lanthanum, gallium, tellurium, yttrium, bismuth, thallium, indium, gold, scandium, tantalum, vanadium, thorium, uranium, samarium, beryllium, tungsten

As you can see from the chart, the human body is made up of mostly oxygen. However, our bodies, like the body of planet Earth, became one big body of water when oxygen and hydrogen merged in a particular way, making our bodies approximately 75% water (H_2O). To better understand the importance of water, its ecology and how the life of that ecology remains sustainably healthy and alive, let's explore together the root meaning of the word hydrogen.

Hydro comes from a Greek word meaning, water. And gen comes from a Greek word meaning, to be born. Thus, the word hydrogen translates, "to be born of water."

When we think about maintaining the ecological health of a body of water, as in a lake or a swimming pool, the first factor to always consider is its pH. In scientific terms, pH stands for potential of Hydrogen, or we could say, potential of water.

Water, by weight, is mostly oxygen and oxygen is the key to life.

The term "pH" is a method of measurement using a scale of numbers to determine the acidity or alkalinity of various substances and solutions, such as water. It's much like using a thermometer to measure your temperature.

The pH scale runs from 0-14. Water with a pH measurement of 0-7 is acid—the closer to zero, the more acidic the water. A pH measurement of 7.0 is defined as neutral, being neither acid nor alkaline. Any number greater than 7.0 is alkaline—the higher the number the greater the alkalinity.

PH-SCALE							
ACID			⟵		⟶	ALKALINE	
TOTAL	VERY	MODERATE	SLIGHT	BALANCE	SLIGHT	MODERATE	VERY EXTREME
0	1-2	3-4	5-6	7	8-9	10-11	12-14

Throughout these chapters, the two most important factors to keep in mind are: (1) if the pH balance of a body of water, as in a lake or swimming pool, is not maintained and the water becomes overly acidic, algae over grows, the water becomes infested with pathogenic bacteria and becomes unfit for humans, fish or cells to swim in and (2) the more acidic the water becomes, the lower the oxygen becomes. And keep in mind that water, by weight, is made up of mostly oxygen and oxygen is the key to a vibrant, healthy life.

HOW BODIES OF WATER DIE

The earth is composed of vast waterways that run through towns and cities. We depend upon these great bodies of water and their tributaries for drinking water, irrigating crops, transporting commodities from one place to another and being a powerful energy source for hydroelectric plants. For communities to thrive, the ecological health of these waterways is extremely important. To understand how the ecology of a waterway can be destroyed, even to the point of death, let's consider what happened to one of our greatest bodies of water, Lake Erie.

Lake Erie, one of the Great Lakes of Canada and the United States, was thriving and replete with ecological life until industrial plants slowly began to surround the lake and began consistently dumping toxic chemicals such as phosphates from sewage treatment plants into its waters. In the early 1970s, Lake Erie became so polluted from chemical dumping that the Environmental Protection Agency (EPA) pronounced it dead.

Most researchers blamed the death of Lake Erie on the overgrowth of algae, which depleted the water's oxygen levels and in turn killed the fish that swam in its waters. Other researchers blamed the dying fish on an infestation of bacteria. However, I believe that the problem originated with the random dumping of toxic chemicals, especially phosphates. Here's why.

A phosphate, an inorganic chemical, is a salt of phosphoric acid, which is highly acidic. Algae, a significant inherent aspect of water ecology, overgrew in its innate attempt to clean up the highly acidic chemicals that threatened the life of the lake. Nature is prolife and constantly strives to sustain ecological balance. Unfortunately, algae requires oxygen for its growth process. The more chemicals that were dumped into the lake, the more the algae overgrew to clean up the chemicals; the more the algae overgrew, the less oxygen in the lake and, the more acidic the water became, the lower the oxygen became.

Because the water's oxygen levels became extremely low, the fish became oxygen-starved, which made it difficult for them to live. Over time, the fish lost their immunity and became diseased and infected with pathogenic bacteria, which are, in essence, reducer organisms. Consequently, the fish began to die in massive numbers.

To compound an already compromised situation, Lake Erie's waters became so polluted with petroleum-based sludge and the gaseous products of rot and fermentation that the

> *Where there is living, oxygen-rich water, there is life. Where there is stagnant, oxygen-starved water, there is death.*

surface of the lake actually caught fire. Dead bloated fish were said to have exploded as they rose to the surface. Johnny Carson joked that Lake Erie was simply a place where fish that had a death urge went to die.

Fortunately, after the EPA forced shoreline industries to drastically reduce their acidifying chemical dumping frenzy by 80%, the lake, over time, restored itself.

HOW THE HUMAN BODY DIES

Since the human body, like the earth, is made up of mostly water and water is made up of mostly oxygen, Lake Erie's fate is a perfect metaphor for understanding how the human body becomes diseased and dies.

Like the earth, our bodies have an intricate circulatory system made up of a complex network of various sized tributaries that run through our towns (glands) and cities (organs) called veins, arteries and capillaries. Like the earth's waterways, these tributaries are designed to transport commodities such as oxygen and vital nutrients from one place to another as well as being a powerful source of electrical energy for every cell of our body.

For our towns (glands) and cities (organs) to thrive, ecological balance of these waterways must be maintained. A sustainable internal community, thriving and replete with life is everything. Like the trillions of fish that swim throughout the waters of the earth, we too have trillions of cells that swim throughout the waters of our body. In fact, water not only flows everywhere outside of us, it flows inside of us, circulating in and out of every little nook and crevice. Water is inside the cell and outside the cell. Our bodies are, in fact, one massive network of waterways.

The sustainability of our internal waterways is based on the electrolyte-mineral composition and quantity of water our cells are swimming in, which include blood, lymph, gastric juices, etc. When our waters are alkaline and electrolyte-mineral-rich and free of toxic waste, our cells flourish. But when our waters are acid and electrolyte-mineral-poor and full of toxic waste, our cells die at an alarming rate and our waterways become conducive to the overgrowth of yeast, which is a unicellular fungi similar to algae.

Like algae in a lake, yeast lives within the human ecology and generally causes no problems. It does, however, have the ability to morph (change its form) to an invasive multi-cellular form known as Candida.

While Candida can be caused by an imbalance of friendly bacteria in the intestinal tract, it can also be caused by blood sugar disorders.

According to Dr. Doug Graham, author of *The 80-10-10 Diet,* Candida is a microbe that lives in the bloodstream and is inherently designed to be there in a regulated fashion moderated by our blood sugar. Candida lives on blood sugar and when our blood sugar is present in normal amounts, the amount of Candida remains stable. The problem arises when blood sugar becomes excessive and Candida is forced to multiply to keep up with the excessive sugar. If a person's insulin is unable to escort the excessive sugar out of the bloodstream, the sugar can't get out and Candida keeps blooming. What keeps the insulin from escorting sugar out is the over consumption of fat—the more fat (especially bad fats like saturated and trans fat) in your diet, the less effective insulin is at getting sugar out of the blood stream. Thus, the over consumption of fat is similar to industry dumping large amounts of petroleum into our earth's waterways.

> *Research has shown that uptake, transport and delivery of sugar is compromised as fat intake rises.*

The long-term danger of Candida overgrowth is a compromised immune system which makes us vulnerable to almost every disease known, which is an underlying ecological debilitation in which most never uncover the underlying cause. In fact, it has recently been discovered that one of our nation's most feared diseases and leading causes of death—cancer—spawns out of this sort of ecological breakdown, a Candida infestation gone wild, caused by an overly acidic pH and decreased oxygen levels.

Several physicians, past and present, have well documented this fact. Today, researcher and oncologist Tullio Simoncini, M.D. of Rome, Italy, has discovered that cancer is a *fungus,* specifically, Candida. In his book, *Cancer is a Fungus,* Dr. Simoncini states, "My idea is that cancer doesn't depend on mysterious causes such as genetic, immunological or auto-immunological as the official oncology proposes, but it comes down from a simple fungal infection."

While deemed unconventional by his colleagues, Dr. Simoncini's method of reversing cancer is as simple, inexpensive and noninvasive as using a highly alkaline substance called bicarbonate of soda (baking soda) injected into the infected area along with a recommended diet high in alkaline foods and low in acid foods. Alkaline foods include plant foods such as fruits and vegetables while acid foods include animal foods such as fish, meat and meat products, milk and dairy products. Acid foods also include most grains and processed foods loaded with toxic chemicals.

As far back as 1924, Dr. Otto Warburg, Doctor of Chemistry and twice Nobel laureate, reported in his research that cancer is caused by the fact that tumor cells mainly generate energy by the breakdown of glucose. He said, "Cancer, above all diseases, has countless secondary causes. But even for cancer, there is only one prime cause. Summarized in a few words, the prime cause of cancer is the replacement of the respiration of oxygen in normal body cells by a fermentation of sugar."

Much of Otto Warburg's original work was published in *The Metabolism of Tumours* and the *New Methods of Cell Physiology*. He wrote about oxygen's relationship to the pH of cancer cells' internal environment. Since fermentation was a major metabolic pathway of cancer cells, he reported that cancer cells maintain a lower pH, as low as 6.0, due to lactic acid production and elevated carbon dioxide (CO_2).

Warburg firmly believed that there was a direct relationship between pH and oxygen. Higher pH means higher concentration of oxygen molecules while lower pH means lower concentrations of oxygen. He demonstrated that all forms of cancer are characterized by two basic conditions: acidosis and hypoxia (lack of oxygen). He stated that a lack of oxygen and acidosis are two sides of the same coin: where you have one you have the other.

To further substantiate this fact, Dr. Sam Whang, in his book, *Reverse Aging,* states that there is a major difference in oxygen levels, even within the narrow range of normal blood pH. He states that when blood has a pH of 7.3, it actually has 69.4% less oxygen than blood that has a perfect pH of 7.45.

In his later years, Dr. Warburg was so convinced that disease resulted from an internal pollution that he became what some would call a health nut because he would only eat organically-grown whole foods. When frustrated by the lack of acceptance of his so-called far-out ideas, Warburg was known to quote a cliché to his colleagues that he attributed to Max Planck, who was honored with The Nobel Prize in Physics, 1918: "science doesn't progress because scientists change their minds, but rather because scientists attached to erroneous views die and are then replaced."

Here's what a few more highly acclaimed medical experts have to say about the health hazards of an overly acidic condition.

> W. F. Koch, M.D., Ph.D. says, *"A cell that has not been starved of oxygen and has a perfect pH balance cannot become infected with cancer."*

> In 1933, William Howard Hay, M.D., published his groundbreaking book, *A New Health Era*. After citing voluminous research, Dr. Hay concluded, *"All disease is caused by auto-intoxication (self-poisoning) due to acid accumulation in the body."*

> Dr. George W. Crile (1864-1943), the father of physiologic surgery, formally recognized as the first surgeon to have succeeded in a direct blood transfusion, and co-founder of the world-famous Cleveland Clinic, stated, *"There is no such thing as natural death. All deaths from so-called natural causes are merely the endpoint of progressive acid saturation."*

> Noted German scientist and microbiologist, Dr. Gunther Ederline (1872-1968), discovered that, "disease cannot survive in an alkaline state," and "total healing only takes place when and if the blood is restored to a normal, slightly alkaline pH."

> Renowned heart specialist and Nobel Prize nominee, Dr. Berthold Kern (1911-1995), was the first to discover that heart infarct (tissue death due to a local lack of oxygen) is caused by metabolic acidosis (over-acidity),

and is nothing but a "gigantic acid catastrophe." Dr. Kern's remedy was the restoration of pH balance to the heart muscle.

Dr. Arthur C. Guyton, M.D., in his book, "The Textbook on Medical Physiology" states, *"All chronic pain, suffering, and diseases are caused by a lack of oxygen (excess acidity at the cell level)."*

Dr. Stephen Levine, renowned Molecular Biologist and Geneticist Author, in his work, "Oxygen Deficiency: A Concomitant to all Degenerative Illness" states, *"In all serious disease states we find a concomitant low oxygen state…low oxygen in the body tissues is a sure indicator for disease…Hypoxia, or lack of oxygen in the tissues, is the fundamental cause for all degenerative disease."*

As you can see, these highly acclaimed medical experts all agree with Béchamp's *Internal Terrain Theory*. As such, there is almost a 100% certainty that anyone living in the Western World is likely to be over-acidic. It has been shown that you are most likely acidic if you consume mostly a typical, Standard American Diet (SAD) of acid-forming foods: meats, cheeses, pasta, refined sugar, fast foods, starches, artificial sweeteners; drink alcohol, coffee, tap water, tea, or sodas; take any prescription drugs, most of the over-the-counter drugs, and many well-known vitamin supplements; or are under stress.

> *Candida is a part of nature's food chain. They are reducer organisms and the bottom line is: if you feed 'em, they'll come!*

The result is, our pH becomes overly acidic, our oxygen levels lower and we become a fertile breeding ground for yeast, bacteria, viruses, parasites, and every manner of pathogenic microorganisms. In other words, disease stems from an "ecological breakdown." All of these microorganisms are a part of nature's food chain. They are reducer organisms and the bottom line is this: if you feed 'em, they'll come!

To begin the *Get Clean Go Green EcoDiet* process of restoring ecological health back into the waters of your body, all you have to do is follow the same instructions the

EPA used to clean up Lake Erie; that is, to simply reduce the amount of acidifying foods and substances you're feeding into your water's ecology by 80%. If you do, over time, your body will have the potential to heal itself and regain its natural vitality. This is because an alkaline environment replete with oxygen is a place where ecological breakdowns cannot exist.

CHAPTER FOUR

Internal Acid Rain

Let's consider yet another way our internal and external environment suffers from chemical pollution and over-acidification: acid rain.

It's a well-known fact that acid rain causes widespread degradation. Acid rain is created when acidic chemicals and toxic by-products are released into the atmosphere from certain commercial and agricultural practices, as well as the burning of fossil fuels such as natural gas, coal and oil. These pollutants react in the atmosphere with water, oxygen and other chemicals and form various compounds, resulting in an acidic residue or "ash" that can be carried through the atmosphere for hundreds of miles from its origin. As moisture condenses around the ash, these compounds return to the earth by way of rain, snow or fog. The effect is acid rain—a condensation that has a pH level of less than 5.5.

When you look at acid rain, it doesn't look any different from normal rain. But as it falls onto the earth, it harms everything it touches. For instance, if acid rain falls into a body of water such as a lake, it makes the lake more acidic. If the pH of water ever drops between 4.5-5.5, aquatic life is challenged, and if it drops below 4.5, nothing can survive.

THE HARMFUL EFFECTS OF ACID RAIN

A tree has a trunk, branches and foliage, which are insulated with a waxy protective coating essential to the tree's immunity. When acid rain falls on a tree, it eats away at its waxy protective coating, exposing its previously protected limbs to the elements, creating a breakdown process called oxidation. The tree then begins to lose its immunity.

A tree has a root system, which has tiny hairs that are responsible for extracting, absorbing and transferring nutrients into the tree. There are billions of microbes that live within the ecology of the soil whose job it is to break down biodegradable matter into absorbable nutrients, forming the basis of the tree's food chain. As acid rain falls to the ground, the microbes are destroyed, thus they are no longer able to do their job.

Heavy metals such as aluminum, mercury, and cadmium, which are normally bound to the soil, become released by the overly acidic condition. These toxic metals, now loosened, are absorbed through the tiny hairs of the tree's root system. This slowly builds up, blocking the flow of other vital nutrients and poisoning the tree. The tree's root system begins to break down, which causes soil to build up inside the root. The tree loses its immunity; it begins to rot and decay.

Reducer organisms like bacteria, yeast, fungus and mold, previously held in check by the immunity of the tree, arrive on the scene to assist nature in returning that which is no longer vital back into the dust of the earth.

Internal Acid Rain & Neurological Diseases

Acid rain is formed within our internal environment in much the same way it is formed within our outer environment. It is created when we burn the wrong types of food for fuel. This is how I believe it happens.

Food is broken down in the digestive tract and used as fuel through various metabolic processes. One of those processes is called oxidation, a chemical reaction whereby oxygen binds itself to an element or compound and then is used by the body as fuel. What is not used for fuel leaves a residue known as ash. This residue, depending on what types of foods are consumed, leaves either an acid ash or an alkaline ash. Thus, these foods are either considered acid ash-forming or alkaline-forming. But for the purpose of simplifying the terminology of these foods, for the rest of the book, I will use acid-forming and alkaline-forming foods instead.

When acid-forming foods are eaten, an internal acid-rain-like acid is formed as bodily fluids condense, or surround themselves, around the acidic ash. This condensation can have a pH level of 5.5 or lower. The ash then travels throughout our internal environment via the blood and cerebrospinal fluid (our body's waterways), depositing its destructive residue throughout our inner ecology—just like acid rain in the outer environment.

Like a tree, we, too, have a trunk called a torso. And just as a tree has its bark, we have skin. The torso houses our spinal column, which is often referred to as the body's "tree of life." The nerves that branch off our tree of life are its branches, and our organs are their fruit. Just as the tree's foliage has a waxy protective covering which shields it from the elements, our nerves have a fatty protective coating known as the myelin sheath, which is essential for covering the nerve's electrical wiring.

Ecological breakdowns occur as a result of an internal acid rain.

In the same manner that acid rain destroys the protective coating on the branches of a tree, the same process takes place within us as the downpour of acid rain burns away at the protective fatty myelin sheath around the nerves. Our tree of life thus loses its immunity and becomes the tree of death. Reducer organisms, such as bacteria, arrive on the scene to reduce what is no longer vital back into the dust of the earth.

This ecological degradation, caused by an acidic-like-rainwater, results in neurological diseases, such as dementia, multiple sclerosis, Alzheimer's, and Parkinson's.

I call this hypothesis *the internal acid rain theory.*

To validate this theory, in 1998, Lorne Label, M.D., conducted several internal terrain pH studies on his patients who had been stricken with neurological diseases. He performed these studies after he and I began having an in-depth conversation about my insights on pH, internal acid rain and the brain terrain. He discussed with me that the latest medical research revealed that *Chlamydia* bacteria could be the cause of these devastating diseases, as they were almost always present in those suffering with Parkinson's, Alzheimer's and multiple sclerosis.

Agreeing that bacteria were opportunistic and most likely not the originating cause of these diseases, he decided to perform spinal taps on some of his patients, since the cerebral spinal fluid is, in effect, the brain's water supply and should reflect a pH value of approximately 7.4.

About a month later, he reported back.

"After contemplating your internal acid rain theory, I performed a number of spinal taps on Alzheimer's, Parkinson's and multiple sclerosis patients, as the cerebral spinal fluid is, in effect, the brain's water supply and should have a pH value of approximately 7.4. When I tested the cerebrospinal fluid's pH, to my amazement, you were right: it was approximately 5.5—the pH of environmental acid rain. Further dietary research is justified to see if shifting the pH of the brain terrain will provide clues in turning these devastating diseases around. From the evidence I now see I am optimistic."

– Lorne Label, M.D.
Doctor of Neurology

Internal Acid Rain & Intestinal Diseases

Like a tree, we, too, have a root system: our intestinal tract. Like the fine hairs on the outside of a root, our intestines have fine hairs on the inside called, villi. Thus, you could say that our intestines are like an inverted root system. Villi, like the fine hairs on a tree's root system, are responsible for extracting, absorbing and transferring nutrients from one part of the body to another.

Heavy metals, which are similarly bound within the mucus of the colon, are harmless until rendered soluble with the saturation of acid rain. When liberated, heavy metals plug up our villi, inhibiting the uptake of nutrients and destroying our immunity (research has recently revealed that 80% of our immune system lies in our gastrointestinal tract).

There are billions of microbes (friendly and unfriendly bacteria) that exist within the ecology of our intestinal tract. Their job, like the microbes within the soil of the earth, is to break down biodegradable matter into absorbable nutrients. These microbes are destroyed by a diet high in acid ash-forming foods.

Like the root of the tree, when the constant downpour of acid rain challenges the root system of our body's tree of life, it becomes clogged with mucus, which is secreted in large quantities in order to afford protection against the acids. This in turn causes our digestive tract to weaken and become even more toxic. Because of this ecological breakdown, the body's entire immune system is significantly impaired and loses its ability to maintain homeostasis. If this condition is allowed to persist, symptoms such as constipation, Candida, leaky gut, irritable bowel syndrome, Crohn's disease, diverticulitis, or colon cancer can result.

This ecological breakdown spirals downward even further when reducer organisms, which are a necessary part of nature's clean-up crew, arrive on the scene to break down what is no longer vital back into the dust of the earth.

So instead of asking how to get rid of the bugs we call our enemy, perhaps we should ask, *why has this enemy arrived on the scene?*

"If I could live my life over again, I would devote it to proving that germs seek their natural habitat—diseased tissue—rather than being the cause of the diseased tissue; e.g., mosquitoes seek the stagnant water, but do not cause the pool to become stagnant."

–Rudolph Virchow, M.D., Ph.D., (1821-1902)

THE FOUR STAGES OF ACIDIFICATION

Acidification of our internal terrain occurs whenever a diet high in acid-forming foods is consumed. Other contributors include negative thoughts and emotions, the use of personal care or household cleaning products loaded with toxic chemicals, toxic indoor air, little or no exercise, lack of rest, shallow breathing and lack of sunshine. Another major factor is not consuming enough of the right kind of water—water that has the ability to facilitate adequate nutrient absorption and efficient disposal of toxic waste. Any single aspect or a combination of any of these conditions generate and accelerate deterioration of our internal environment.

As I see it, the development of acidification progresses through four distinctive stages of degradation as follows:

Stage 1

The first stage of disease is a process known as autointoxication. It forms whenever acid-forming foods are fed into the internal environment of the body. Over time, as the acidic waste accumulates, the blood stream becomes congested, which slows down circulation. Decreased circulation affects our blood's ability to effectively transport oxygen and other vital nutrients to the trillions of cells that swim within our watery terrain. It also interferes with immune cells in our blood.

As acidic waste continues to accumulate, our organs of elimination (bowel, lungs, skin, kidneys), and the liver, become increasingly more sluggish and ineffective because the body is forced to continually protect itself against acids by creating a sticky mucus-like waste. Our internal waterways become more and more acidic and this mucus-like waste gets deposited wherever it can, i.e., skin, various organs, and glands. Gradually, our energy decreases and the body struggles to maintain ecological balance. Our towns (glands) and cities (organs) begin to lose their electrical potential. This toxic overload produces the first stage of yeast overgrowth, symptoms we label colds, flu, various aches and pains and just feeling off center, or out of sorts.

Some of the physical and emotional conditions associated with this first stage of acidification are sluggishness, mild depression, muscle tension, constipation and/or diarrhea, headache, upset stomach, heartburn, sore throat, irritability, skin eruptions, kidney or bladder infection, muscle aches, floating anxiety, hypoglycemia, short attention span, hyperactivity, confusion, sinus pressure, mucous drainage, weight gain or loss, nightmares, hypersensitivity or tendency to overreact, etc. Over time, if these acidic wastes are not properly eliminated, they settle deeper into the tissues, causing chronic or more serious conditions to develop.

Stage 2

The second stage of disease is a process known as auto-immunization. The immune system has now become compromised and unable to prevent the onslaught of microbial invasions. These microbes, which are reducer organisms, come on the scene to do their inherent job of decomposing that which is no longer vital. The further damage that is created by these pathogens in our organs, glands and tissue, triggers an inflammatory response by the immune system in attempt to repair itself. This inflammatory response is how I view the process of internal global warming and the many health crises it causes.

Chronic symptoms progress toward environmental or food allergies, migraine headaches, high blood pressure, irritable bowel syndrome, leaky gut, acid reflux, celiac disease, Crohn's disease, high cholesterol, asthma, sinus infections, lupus, chronic fatigue syndrome, fibromyalgia, kidney stones, gallstones, Parkinson's, Alzheimer's, multiple sclerosis, bronchial pneumonia, depression, obesity, addictions, diabetes, etc.

Stage 3

The third stage of disease is a process known as autoinfection. It takes place when the proliferation of microbial organisms takes place rapidly in a now suitable host. Cell death accelerates and the body is now in a full-blown state of chronic acidosis. Systemic Candida yeast infection rages out of control. The body's ability to adapt becomes overwhelmed in its attempt to sustain ecological balance. If the body's SOS signals are not heeded, the automatic response is unremitting re-infection with larvae produced by parasites and worms. In essence, the undertakers have arrived on the scene.

Some of the physical conditions associated with this advanced stage of acidification are: heart attack, cancer, AIDS and advanced expressions of stage-two conditions.

Stage 4

The fourth and final stage of disease is a process known as auto-predictable death!

If you're presently suffering from any of these various stages of acidification, and you now see that disease is but an ecological breakdown produced by an internal acid rain, maybe you can finally let go of the theory that germs and disease are your enemy and take hold of the truth behind what the philosopher Pogo once said:

…we have met the real enemy and the enemy is us!

CHAPTER FIVE

The Internal Acid Rain Study

Fortunately, there's a way for you to see first-hand that a diet high in processed foods loaded with toxic chemicals and animal protein with their by-products creates acid rain within your internal environment. There's also a way for you to determine the condition of your internal environment and see if the types of food you've been eating have damaged your inner rainforest and depleted your life-giving oxygen.

Is acid rain running through my veins; burning my inner rainforest; depleting my life-giving oxygen?

Like scientists or environmental ecologists who conduct acid rain tests to check the pH levels of acid rain falling within particular geographical regions, you, too, can conduct this same test within your own internal environment. I call it the internal acid rain study.

The analogy is simple: your urine is your body's rainwater.

To perform this internal acid rain study, you can either use litmus paper or pH sticks, which can be found at most health food stores. You may even be inspired to enroll your family or a close friend to take the test with you and compare your scores. It's fun, informative and life changing. Just keep in mind that this pH test is not meant to be a comprehensive diagnostic tool; it is an internal acid rain study only.

You, too, are now on your way to becoming a *Body Ecologist*!

ACID & ALKALINE FOODS

Before beginning your environmental study, it's important to review the acid-alkaline food chart below, as it will greatly assist you with your food choices while performing the acid rain study. Keep in mind that if a food increases the acidity of urine, it is classified as an acid-forming food. Conversely, if a food increases the alkalinity of urine, it is classified as an alkaline-forming food.

Below is a summary of which foods are the most and the least acid-forming and which ones are the most and the least alkaline-forming.

Strong Acid-Forming Foods	Mild Acid-Forming Foods
Red Meat	Grains
Pork	Beans
Chicken	Legumes
Eggs	Nuts
Dairy	Seeds
Processed Foods	Fish

Strong Alkaline-Forming Foods	Mild Alkaline-Forming Foods
Wheatgrass	Fruits
Green Leafy Vegetables	Vegetables
Green Juices & Powders	Sea Vegetables

Note All organic, unrefined cold-pressed fats and oils have a neutral pH, being neither acid nor alkaline. Generally speaking, foods that have been altered from their natural form are acid-forming.

HOW TO TEST YOUR pH

To begin, before making any changes to your diet, eat the foods you would normally eat for 24 hours. This will give you a baseline reading. Thus, you'll be able to chart your results as change evolves and ecological balance is restored.

Day 1—Baseline Test

Eat the foods you would normally eat for one entire day (24 hours). Before going to bed, place a disposable cup next to your commode. The next morning upon waking, collect your first morning urine. Dip the pH stick in the urine and shake off the excess. Compare the color with the color chart and record your results. Depending on what you ate and your body's ability to buffer acids, your measurement should read between 5.5 and 8.0. If you ate mostly acid-forming foods the previous day, your pH should read between 5.8 and 6.0. If you've eaten mostly alkaline-forming foods, your pH should read between 6.4 and 6.8.

Day 2—Acid Meal Test

To perform the internal acid rain study, devote one entire day (24 hours) to eating only acid-forming foods such as meat, pasta, beans, bread, nuts, fish, dairy, and eggs. If you're already a vegetarian or vegan, just eat foods that are mildly acid-forming such as grains and beans. Have no alkaline-forming foods at all...no vegetables, fruits or their juices. Upon waking the next morning, repeat the urine test. If your buffering mechanism is functioning at its greatest capacity and your alkaline reserves have not been exhausted, your urine should reflect the ash from the foods eaten the day before, which is acid. Thus, a healthy pH reading would be 4.5-5.5—the pH of acid rain.

Day 3—Alkaline Meal Test

Devote one entire day (24 hours) to eating only alkaline-forming foods such as fruits and vegetables and their juices. Have no acid ash-forming foods at all: no grains, beans, chemicalized processed foods, dairy, meat, coffee or tea (refer to the acid list given). You will also want to exclude any vitamins or minerals you are presently taking. Upon waking the next morning, repeat the urine test. If your buffering mechanism is functioning at its greatest capacity and your alkaline reserves have not been exhausted, your urine should reflect the ash from the foods eaten the day before, which is alkaline. Thus, a healthy pH reading would be 7.0.

The section below will greatly assist you in understanding more about pH readings, alkaline reserves and buffering. For a more in-depth understanding, I recommend Dr. Ted Morter, Jr.'s book, *Correlative Urinalysis* or *Your Health Your Choice*.

ELECTROLYTES, POTENTIAL & BUFFERING

Adequate electrolytes are absolutely essential for the life and health of our bodies. If we become even slightly deficient in electrolytes, we lose our health and if we run too long, our bodies cannot survive. Though there are numerous life-essential functions involving electrolytes, the three most important are: (1) to provide the electrical continuity of our cells, (2) to provide the components of the sodium-potassium pump that moves food into the cell and waste out and (3) to help maintain the proper acid-alkaline balance.

Sodium, potassium, calcium, magnesium, lithium, and phosphorus are the main electrolytes the body requires for almost every bodily function, making it imperative for electrolyte balance to be maintained. If a slight depletion of electrolytes occur, organs become severely challenged, weakened, toxic, and sluggish, which can also cause extreme alterations in the rates of chemical reactions—inside and outside of our cells. Any depletion of electrolytes means acids are increasing and the body is losing control, which means our health is moving in a downward cycle and healing is significantly inhibited.

Electrolytes are the ionic compounds in water that provide it with the ability to carry an electrical charge. In essence, they are catalyst for electrical potential, and the human body is a fine-tuned electrically charged instrument. In fact, every cell of your body is electrical. Cells operate much like a power plant, or better yet, like the battery that starts your automobile. An electrochemical battery, or more precisely, a cell, is any device in which the reaction between two substances can be made to occur in such a way that some of the chemical energy is converted to useful electricity.

If acids are allowed to accumulate around your vehicle's battery cable, much like the membrane around your cells, your battery cable (cell membrane) becomes hardened and impermeable, lowering the voltage within your cells, decreasing their potential to jump start your engine. And without proper electrical flow, the cell's ability to efficiently absorb nutrients and eliminate acid waste begins to decline.

Electrolytes are the primary component for maintaining a healthy blood pH of 7.35-7.45. If our fluids start to run low in electrolytes, which is mostly due to a diet high in acid-forming foods, the human body has a built-in mechanism or "mechanic" to make sure the blood pH stays in its very narrow range. This mechanism is called buffering, a necessary course of action that keeps our engine running.

Buffering is our body's way of protecting us against acidosis and alkalosis. While there are several buffering systems for different bodily functions, sodium bicarbonate is our first line of defense against excessive acid build-up. The downside is that, if our buffering mechanism is forced to pull electrolytes from our alkaline reserves day in and day out, year after year without adequate replenishment of electrolytes, we eventually run out of alkaline reserves.

Alkaline reserves is a term that reflects the amount of buffering compounds, i.e. sodium bicarbonate in the blood capable of neutralizing acids. A healthy body generally has a large amount of alkaline reserves (buffering compounds), which are used to meet any emergency demands. The downside is that if our alkaline reserves start to run low, our lungs and kidneys become overwhelmed with acid waste, and acid deposits begin to accumulate in the weaker tissues or organs of our body. Then, if our alkaline reserves become exhausted, our bodies are equipped with a last resort emergency back-up system. This buffer is called ammonia.

Ammonia is highly alkaline, having a pH of approximately 10.5. As a point of reference, if you've ever walked into a nursing home and smelled a strong scent of ammonia, know that the odor is *not* coming from the cleaning crew's mop bucket. It's coming from the ammonia-riddled urine of the elderly in their last days, which is a sure sign that their alkaline reserves have been completely exhausted and their buffering mechanism is using ammonia as a last ditch effort to buffer the acids and keep them alive.

This is why, when conducting the internal acid rain study and eating only acid-forming foods for 24 hours, if your pH numbers are higher than 6.0, it's a sure sign that your alkaline reserves are low and alkaline reserves become low when your body runs low in electrolytes.

If your pH numbers are higher than 7.5, it's a sure sign that your body is in the ammonia cycle to help deal with the acid. Likewise, when eating only alkaline-forming foods for 24 hours, if your pH numbers are lower than 7.0, it is also a sure sign that your alkaline reserves are low. But not to worry–there *is* an answer. The answer to building up your alkaline reserves and preventing or reversing a type of ecological breakdown is *electrolytes*.

Electrolytes are the key to turning your environmental crisis around.

Electrolytes are the alkaline salts in the body that conduct every electrical cellular activity, and are only available in adequate amounts when you eat a plant-based alkaline diet.

So if you're ready to turn your environmental crisis around and live the vibrant, healthy life you were designed to live, then stop acidifying your environment and start alkalizing. If you do, every cell of your body will become like an alkaline battery so you, too, can keep going on and on and on and on…

CHAPTER SIX

Stop Acidifying & Start Alkalizing!

If you're presently experiencing an ecological breakdown and you've just discovered that *acid rain is running through your veins*...or you simply want to become a *Body Ecologist* and prevent it, then it's time to heed your body's SOS signal and "Answer the Call."

The SOS signal is sounding $\cdots$ $-$ $-$ $-$ $\cdots$ so let's decipher what I believe the signal is saying:

Stop burning the wrong types of salt, oil and sugar into your internal environment!

S–O–S
Salt–Oil–Sugar

Almost every processed food that sits on your grocery store shelves is not only preserved with toxic chemicals that acidify your environment and affect the health of your ecology, it is also loaded with the wrong type of salt, oil and sugar. Even though salt, oil and sugar do not leave an acid "ash," these substances are still among the top three acidifiers of the body and are, unfortunately, heavily featured among those who are eating the Standard American Diet (SAD). With this in mind, it's not too difficult to understand why the U.S. Department of Health in 1982, ranked America to be one of the sickest of 100 civilized nations on earth. America ranked 95th in relation to chronic and degenerative diseases; only five countries were worse off than America. In 1987, it was revealed that America had dropped to the bottom of the list—number 100.

The Wrong Type of Salt

If the salt (or the processed food that contains it) in your pantry has been refined, throw it out! The wrong type of salt to your cells is like too much sunlight to a grape. While salt is essential for life, the wrong type of salt dehydrates your cells and lowers their electrical potential, and thus lowering your potential to achieve optimal health and a state of wellbeing.

There's an enormous difference between refined salt most people are accustomed to using and a whole food salt. Refined table salt is actually 97.5% sodium chloride and 2.5% chemicals such as moisture absorbents and iodine. Dried at over 1,200°F, the excessive heat substantially alters the natural chemical structure of the salt, no matter if it's land salt or sea salt. What remains after most salts are chemically cleaned is sodium chloride, an unnatural form of salt that your body identifies as something completely foreign. Essential minerals and trace elements were removed as impurities. Refined salt often contains potentially harmful preservatives such as aluminum hydroxide to prevent clumping. This form of unnatural salt has earned the name "white poison."

The body isolates excess salt by *extracting water from your cells* to neutralize the unnatural sodium chloride. The resulting consequence is a less-than-ideal fluid balance. For every gram of sodium chloride your body cannot get rid of, 23 times that amount of cell water is used to neutralize the salt. Thus, refined salt causes excess fluid build up, which can contribute to unsightly cellulite, along with rheumatism, arthritis, gout, kidney stones, and gallstones.

Regrettably, refined salt not only sits on most every kitchen table across our nation, it is found in almost every processed product that you eat. When you consider that the average person consumes 4,000 to 6,000 milligrams of sodium chloride each day, and heavy users can ingest as much as 10,000 milligrams in a day, it is clear that this is a serious and pervasive issue. In fact, most researchers and physicians across the world have found that a diet high in sodium chloride contributes to a number of health risks such as high blood pressure, heart disease, stroke, and certain kinds of cancers. Still, salt is as fundamental to our life as air and water, and without it we could not exist.

The Right Type of Salt

In ancient times, salt was considered more valuable than gold. In those days, salt was considered the fifth element because its qualities are comparable only to ether.

The human body is primarily made of water and salt. The relationship between water and salt is what makes our heart beat, the synapses in our brain function, our tendons move, and our nerves send messages to our brain. The crystalline nature of salt is the stored information that rebuilds our DNA, which in turn has the potential to reconstruct our body and mind back into our original nature. To be called "The Salt of the Earth" is to be considered a good person.

The brand I recommend is Celtic Sea Salt®. Celtic Sea Salt® is harvested off the coast of France using methods originating with the Celts many centuries ago, leaving it in its natural crystal form. The natural methods used to harvest this particular brand of sea salt enable the crystals to maintain not only a wonderful, clean flavor, but the diverse amount of healthy minerals craved by the human body remain inherent within the salt as well.

Celtic Sea Salt® imparts a pure, fresh taste to your meals, rather than the harsh flavor of regular table salt. But more importantly, nearly eighty vital nutrients and minerals can be found in the tiny, gray crystals of Celtic Sea Salt®, serving to provide the body with a healthy dose of electrolytes, energy and other healthy body functions such as immune system strengthening and the absorption of nutritious elements from food. The trace minerals also play an important part in cleansing the body and aiding in healthy digestion. Many health car practitioners like myself include Celtic Sea Salt® in their regular diet, as the balance of minerals and nutrients is an optimum choice for those living a healthy lifestyle.

When mixed with water, these salts offer us the best in most every natural element known; identical to the 84 elements found in the human body.

Health Benefits of Celtic Sea Salt®:

- Regulates water balance throughout the body.
- Promotes a healthy pH balance in the cells, particularly your brain cells.
- Promotes a healthy blood sugar.
- Helps to reduce signs of aging.
- Assists in the generation of hydroelectric energy in the cells.
- Helps with absorption of food particles throughout the intestinal tract.
- Supports respiratory health.
- Promotes sinus health.
- Prevents muscle cramps.
- Promotes bone strength.
- Regulates sleep patterns.
- Supports libido.
- Promotes vascular health.
- Regulates blood pressure.

The Wrong Type of Oil

If the oil (or the processed food that contain it) in your pantry has been hydrogenated or partially hydrogenated, throw it out! Consuming the wrong type of oil is like dumping petroleum into the earth's waterways. While fats are essential for life, the wrong type of fat suffocates your cells and lowers their electrical potential, and thus your ability to reach optimal health.

The wrong type of fats are saturated and trans fats. Saturated fats raise total blood cholesterol as well as LDL cholesterol (the "bad" cholesterol). Saturated fats are mainly found in animal products such as meat, dairy, eggs, and seafood. Trans fats are the most harmful fats as they are extremely harmful to your arteries and are known to create cardiovascular disease. These unhealthy fats are often found in fast foods such as fried chicken and French fries; junk foods such as doughnuts, cookies, candy bars, potato chips, pastries, and crackers; and in processed staples on the grocery shelves, from soup mixes to margarine.

Trans fats are created through the process of hydrogenation. Hydrogenation is the process by which hydrogen is forced into highly heated vegetable oil with the aid of a catalyst, usually nickel. Forcing hydrogen into the oil changes the chemical structure so that the oil will become more solid. Fully hydrogenating oils makes them too solid, which makes them difficult to use for cooking. Partially hydrogenating oils creates a slightly soft texture, making it the perfect consistency for items such as margarine and shortening. When oils are only partially hydrogenated, the molecules of the partially hydrogenated oils form *trans* configurations, which means the oil molecules have kind of an odd shape for fat molecules. Your body doesn't like this *trans* configuration, making trans fats even more harmful than saturated fats.

Trans fats are known to cause intense free-radical activity. The process of oxidation that occurs in reactions with free radicals can turn cell membranes rancid and stiff. The resulting rigidity impedes the free flow of oxygen through the membrane and interrupts electronic transfers of energy, producing a kind of bioelectrical short. Trans fats also interfere with the circulation of oxygen in the blood, creating a state of acidosis.

Needless to say, trans fats are associated with the common degenerative diseases that kill Western populations. In one of many examples of warnings, a Harvard review of evidence verifies that eating trans fats increases the risk of heart disease. A Harvard School of Public Health press release on June 12, 1999, revealed that "...if trans fats were replaced by unsaturated vegetable oils, we would expect to see at least 30,000 fewer persons die prematurely from coronary heart disease each year." That number was based on the United States alone.

Be aware that according to FDA guidelines, products containing less than 0.5g trans fat per serving can list zero grams trans fat on their nutritional labels. As a result, just one "zero grams trans fat" serving could contain as much as 0.49g of trans fat. Over the course of three meals—breakfast, lunch and dinner—just one serving of "zero grams trans fat" at each meal can add up to almost 1.5g of trans fat per day.

Another unhealthy oil to watch out for is canola oil. Oils, such as olive oil come from olives, peanut oil come from peanuts and sunflower oil come from sunflowers. But have you ever wondered where canola oil comes from? Canola is a genetically engineered plant developed in Canada from the Rapeseed plant, which is part of the mustard family of plants—a toxic and poisonous weed which, when processed, becomes rancid very quickly. According to an article written in *The Wall Street*

Journal on June 7, 1995, canola oil has been shown to cause lung cancer in humans. Some writer/researchers report that canola oil was never designed for human consumption; that it has long been used by small industries as a lubricating agent and is also an excellent insect repellent. But, according to Mary G. Enig, Ph.D. and Director of Nutritional Sciences Division, the major problem with canola oil is that it has to be partially hydrogenated or refined before it can be used commercially and consequently is a source of trans fats, sometimes at very high levels.

Another consideration is oils that have been bottled in clear bottles and stored in the light for a long periods of time where they are subject to oxidation and rancidity. Rancid oils can generally be recognized by flavor and smell.

The Right Type of Oil

Even though vegetable oils tend to have a neutral pH, being neither acid nor alkaline, they definitely have an alkalizing effect on the body. So, when you're "chewing the fat," make sure you're chewing the right fat. Fats that naturally occur in plant foods are the fats that sustain us and heal us when we're ill. In fact, Dr. Udo Erasmus, renowned authority on fats and human nutrition and author of *Choosing the Right Fats,* says that fats are the most important nutrients known, even more important than vitamins, minerals, or even proteins. The reason is, without them, the very foundation of life energy is lost.

When choosing the right fats, choose plant fats. They contain fatty acids, which are the active ingredient in every bodily process, including brain cell function, nervous system activity, regulating hormones, intracellular messaging, glandular function, immune system operation and hemoglobin oxygen-transport system. Fatty acids are also crucial for cell wall function (passing oxygen into the cell, passing nutrients into the cell and keeping foreign bodies out of the cell), digestive-tract operation, assimilating nutrients and blocking out allergens.

While the human body manufactures most of the fatty acids needed to sustain life, there are two fats that are considered essential, Omega-3 and Omega-6. Essential means that (unlike Omega-7 and Omega-9) you must get them from outside sources. They are found in the healing oils of freshly pressed almonds, flaxseed, sunflower and sesame seeds, hazelnuts, pumpkin, pistachio, and olives.

According to Dr. Erasmus, the daily consumption of both Omega-3 and Omega-6 in their proper balance is vitally important. He says that we get way too much Omega-6 and far too little Omega-3 fatty acids. But taken in the right amounts and ratios, and taken from the right sources, essential fatty acids establish and maintain health and a sense of wellbeing.

Health Benefits of Essential Fatty Acids:

- Increase energy, performance and stamina. Help build muscle, prevent muscle break down, and speed recovery from fatigue.

- Strengthen the immune system. Make hormones that regulate immune and inflammatory responses. Have anti-inflammatory effects and can slow autoimmune damage.

- Lower most risk factors for cardiovascular disease. Lower abnormally high levels of blood pressure, triglycerides, fibrinogen, clot formation, and inflammation.

- Improve brain function, mood, intelligence, behavior and vision. Our brain is over 60% fat. These power omegas are important components of the entire nervous system. They are necessary in the production of serotonin, which helps to prevent depression and other brain diseases.

- Aid in weight reduction. Help keep mood and energy up and suppresses appetite, thereby aiding in weight loss. More recently, they have been found to block the genes that produce fat in the body (saturated and trans fat do not have this same effect) and increase thermo-genesis (heat).

- Regulate organs and glands, such as the liver, kidneys, adrenal and thyroid glands, along with supporting the production of male and female hormones.

- Speed recovery and healing. Necessary for cell growth and division, beginning with the formation of cell membranes; regulate cell activity.

- Support healthy child development. For nervous system development, a growing fetus needs optimum fatty acids from the mother's body. Mothers become depleted of fatty acids during pregnancy, and need optimal fatty acid intake for their own health and their child's optimum development.

- Improve digestion. Poorly digested foods tie up the immune system and can cause gut inflammation, leaky gut, and allergies. They improve gut integrity and decrease inflammation and leaky gut syndrome.

- Decrease infection. Have anti-fungal, anti-yeast, and antimicrobial properties, which helps protect against infections.

- Keep bones strong. Aid in the transport of minerals that keep bones and teeth strong, helping to prevent osteoporosis.

- Protect genetic material. Regulate gene expression, and inhibit tumor growth.

- Ease pre-menstrual syndrome (PMS).

- Produce beautiful skin, hair and nails. Some of the first signs of fatty-acid deficiencies are dry, flaky skin, dull hair, and brittle nails. They help skin conditions such as eczema, psoriasis and acne.

When looking for the best oil blend to consume every day, look for *Udo's Oil 3-6-9 Blend*, derived from organically grown plant sources, found in the cooler section at most health food stores. Use two tablespoons per day every day and observe the results. Just be sure that all the other oils you purchase are organic, cold-pressed and come in dark bottles. A favorite salad oil of mine is Grapeseed Oil, designed by nature to increase the good lipids and reduce the bad ones.

The Wrong Type of Sugar

If the sugar (or the processed food that contain it) in your pantry has been refined, throw it out! The wrong type of sugar to your cells is like pouring espresso into the gas tank of your automobile. While sugar is essential for life, the wrong type of sugar gets your adrenaline revving, which causes you to crash and burn, and too much adrenaline lowers your electrical potential.

According to many holistic physicians, when it comes to the dangerous impact of sugar, "if it's white—it's killing you!" This may sound overly simplistic, but it does sum up the situation when it comes to sugar and its impact on your overall state of wellbeing. It is important to learn about whole food sugars, which can have remarkable health benefits. Refined white sugar, the table sugar that most people use every day, is harmful, even in small amounts.

Until the 1970s, most of the sugar we ate came from sucrose, which is derived from sugar beets or sugar cane. After that, sugars manufactured from corn, such as corn syrup, fructose, dextrose, dextrin, and especially high fructose corn syrup, began to gain popularity as sweeteners because they were much less expensive to produce. According to the Weston Price Foundation, high fructose corn syrup is a highly processed sugar that we should avoid at all cost. High fructose corn syrup can be manipulated to contain equal amounts of fructose and glucose, or up to 80% fructose and 20% glucose. Thus, with almost twice the fructose, *high fructose corn syrup delivers a double-danger* compared to refined white sugar, and it's found in almost every processed food that sits on your grocer's shelves.

Not only is high fructose corn syrup considered one of the major contributors to obesity and type-2 diabetes, a study published in the journal *Environmental Health* in 2009 reported that high fructose corn syrup was commonly tainted with mercury, and found traces of mercury in many common retail products, such as processed foods, that contained high fructose corn syrup as an ingredient. The mercury appears to come from caustic soda and hydrochloric acid, two chemicals used in the manufacture of high-fructose corn syrup that can, depending on their manufacturing process, contains trace amounts of mercury. The Institute for Agriculture and Trade Policy, a nonprofit group based in Minneapolis, Minnesota, tested 55 consumer items, finding mercury in one third of the samples ranging from 30 to 350 parts per trillion. The group said these items included many preferred processed foods by children.

Synthetic sugars such as aspartame (marketed as NutraSweet, Equal and Spoonful) are many times sweeter to the taste than sugar. Aspartame is a protein produced from aspartic acid, an amino acid occurring in many plant proteins that can also be produced by humans and animals. It should be avoided at all cost. When the temperature of aspartame exceeds 86°F, it converts to formaldehyde and then to formic acid, which causes metabolic acidosis. Aspartame is known to change the brain's chemistry, causing severe seizures, neurological diseases, birth defects, memory loss, vertigo, depression, anxiety attacks, and many other known and unknown disorders.

The Right Type of Sugar

Contrary to what you may have been told, some sugars can be healthful like the naturally-occurring sugars in plants such as raw cane, fruits, berries and vegetables. These sugars naturally support your pancreas, your brain, boost your immunity, build and tone your muscles and can even assist you in losing weight. For example, complex sugars found in wolfberries, a Chinese berry also called goji, have been clinically shown to break down tumors, improve eyesight, combat free radicals, strengthen the liver and pancreas, improve weight loss and boost your metabolism. And goji berries have been touted as the greatest antioxidant known.

In fruits and plant foods, sugars are combined with and balanced by other ingredients such as water, vitamins, minerals salts, fiber as well as other beneficial elements known and unknown.

There are many natural sugars, with their nutrients still intact, available at most health food stores, to replace the white sugar you may have been using.

Yacon Syrup is a low-glycemic, low calorie, alternative sweetener that helps strengthen your bones and improves your digestive system. Yacon is known as the richest source of *fructooligosaccharides* (FOS) of any food in the entire world. These long chain sugars help nourish the good bacteria beneficial for digestion. Yacon not only encourages the growth of good bacteria, it also nourishes it so that the body is better able to absorb essential vitamins and minerals. The health benefits are seemingly endless.

Rapadura is a Portuguese name for dehydrated sugarcane juice. It is dried in the form of a brick and is largely produced on sight at sugarcane plantations in very warm tropical regions. This process preserves all of the mineral-rich molasses, particularly silica.

Raw Honey is a honey that has been collected by beekeepers since the dawn of civilization. Aristotle called it "the nectar of the gods." One of the most natural and sustaining of all foods, honey is easy to digest, quickly assimilated into the body, and has a deliciously mild, sweet taste. When used medicinally, raw honey can soothe sore throats and digestive upset, decrease allergy symptoms and, when applied to wounds, it can even kill bacteria and promote healing. Just be sure to purchase it raw and organic.

Date Sugar is an unprocessed sugar made from dehydrated dates that are ground into tiny bits that can be used as a sweetener. Date sugar is high in fiber, with an extremely long list of vitamins and minerals.

Sorghum Syrup is made from sweet sorghum, a grain related to millet that grows on woody stalks to a height of 15 feet. The syrup is made by boiling the sorghum sap. It takes 8-12 gallons of sap to make one gallon of syrup. This highly nutritious sweetener contains B vitamins and minerals like iron, calcium and phosphorus.

Naturally Sweetened Jams and Jellies There are now jams and jellies at most local health food stores sweetened with dehydrated sugarcane juice rather than fructose or high fructose corn syrup. These are the ones with the right type of sugar to put in your grocery cart.

Stevia is a low-calorie sweetener that comes in powder or liquid extract form. It comes from the leaves of several species of plants from the genus *Stevia*. It may be one of the most perfect low-calorie sugar substitutes for the human body because it does not cause an insulin spike. Stevia has been shown to support the function of the pancreas, increasing enzyme availability and improving the body's ability to process other sugars. Sold in the U.S. as a dietary supplement, it can be found in either liquid or powdered form in most health food stores. Like aspartame (one of the most toxic sugar substitutes known to humankind), it is sometimes criticized for its slightly bitter aftertaste. Stevia has also been shown to reduce cavities and has few to no calories.

Organic Zero is a low-calorie organic sugar substitute that has recently hit the market, touted as lacking the aftertaste and digestive side effects of many others. The product has less than one calorie per teaspoon and rates zero on the glycemic index. Made from liquefied organic cane sugar, this product is the perfect substitute for artificial sweeteners. Organic Zero's only ingredient, organic Erythritol, occurs naturally in fermented foods, and many fruits and vegetables. Our own bodies even produce it naturally.

STOP ACIDIFYING!
ACID-FORMING FOODS & DRINKS

While I believe that highly refined salt, oil and sugar and the processed foods that contain them are among the body's top three acidifiers, the foods listed below are also high on the acidifying food chain. Some of these foods are more acidifying than others. The foods listed in the *strong acid-forming food* category are foods that should be completely eliminated from your diet.

The foods listed in the *mild acid-forming food* category are plant-based foods that are needed by the human body, but should only be approximately 20% of your daily diet.

STRONG ACID-FORMING FOODS & DRINKS
(completely eliminate)

Red meat, pork, processed meat, chicken, fish, eggs, dairy,
chemicalized processed foods and drinks

All animal products, red meat, pork, processed meat, chicken, fish, eggs and dairy, even if they are organic, grass-fed or cage-free, are strong acid-forming foods, and should be completely eliminated from your diet. All animal foods create a strong acid ash and, to recap, ash is a metabolic byproduct of digestion. These high protein foods produce strong inorganic acids, such as nitric, sulfuric, and phosphoric, all of which require mineral reserves (electrolytes) such as organic sodium for neutralization. Because it is highly critical that the acid residue of animal proteins be buffered before use and elimination, the body is forced to use its mineral reserves. This is one of the many reasons why meat, even if it is organic and grass-fed, should be completely avoided. Eventually, if too much animal protein is consumed without consuming enough alkaline minerals from plant foods such organic fruits and vegetables, it will deplete the body's alkaline reserves and meat, more than any other acid-forming foods, will do it faster than any other food known.

> **Note** For those of you who do not want to shift to an all plant-based diet or who need more time to transition, eat organic grass-fed meat and organic raw grass-fed dairy products from healthy, happy animals and completely avoid factory-farmed meats, dairy and eggs as they are not environmentally friendly…internally or externally.

Organic animal farming Organic animal farming constitutes the raising of livestock on open pastures and the raising of hens who have plenty of room to do the things that they love most: scratch, flap their wings, perch, nest and roost in a carefully managed, safe, low stress environment—eggs that are free from pesticides, synthetic hormones and animal byproducts. For these animals, there is no caging or confinement and their diet natural to them, which consisting of a variety of grasses, legumes and plants. Research has even shown that grass-fed animals are safer to consume than food from conventionally factory-farmed animals. These animals are not only free of antibiotics, steroids, hormones, pesticides and other foreign substances toxic to their bodies, according to a study published in the *Journal of Animal Science* in 2002, grass-fed beef is lower in fat and calories, has more Omega-3 fatty acids due to the chloroplasts of green leaves and algae they eat, has more vitamins and has as much as 3-5 times more CLA (a newly discovered good fat called "conjugated linoleic acid" that may be a potent cancer fighter) than grain-fed animals.

Factory-farmed animals As stated earlier, animals raised for food production are treated more like commodities than animals. They are handled as units of production, rather than living, breathing creatures. This mechanized approach ignores the needs of animals, which often sacrifices their health and wellbeing in the name of profit. Although there is controversy surrounding the degrees of comfort and freedom that farm animals should have, most agree that farm animals deserve a minimum standard of cleanliness and space, and that animals should not be made to suffer needlessly. While the conditions of these farms range far beyond cruel and unsanitary, most people neglect to explore the far-reaching issues at hand and continue to blindly eat meat and other animal products raised and processed by these inhumane farming methods. Coming face-to-face with these facts isn't always easy.

> ***Cows*** Most male caves are slaughtered at birth and sold for cheap beef, castrated before the age of three months and sent to feedlots to be fattened, or sold to be raised for veal. Female calves, intended for the dairy industry, are separated from their mothers within the first few days of life, moved to a rearing operation where they are fed milk replacer rather than milk, and often have their tails "docked," or cut off. Tail docking is a painful procedure

presumably intended to keep the cow from developing infections caused by constant exposure to manure. However, there is evidence that this practice is simply conducted for the convenience of dairy workers since the lack of a tail provides easier access to the cow's udders. Dairy cows are bred to produce unnaturally large quantities of milk, which weakens their bodies and makes them vulnerable to disease. Cattle in both the beef and dairy industry also show high levels of stress and lameness resulting from the rough manner in which they are handled and their extreme living conditions. Whether on crowded feedlots where animals are exposed to heat and sun or rain, snow, and freezing temperatures, or in tightly packed and unsanitary barns, tethered by short ropes around their necks, the lives of factory farm cattle are marked by physical and mental suffering.

Pigs Factory-farmed pigs are born in small crates that limits their mobility to move around. As the mother lays immobile, unable to make a nest or separate herself and her offspring from their feces, piglets are confined in the crate together, prohibited from running, jumping and playing according to their natural tendencies. Once separated from their mother, pigs are confined together in concrete pens with no bedding or soil for them to root in. In such conditions, pigs become restless and often resort to biting other pig's tails as an expression of stress. Rather than simply giving the pigs straw to play in, many factory farm operators cut off their pig's tails in response to their behavior.

Chickens Chickens raised in large-scale poultry and egg farms are packed individually in cages or all together in large pens; in either case, the average bird spends its entire life in a space smaller than a piece of writing paper. More often than not, they are confined so tightly to wire cages that they cannot stretch their wings, clean themselves, turn around, or exhibit any of their normal behaviors at all. Cages are stacked row upon row inside overheated hangars, which makes these birds subject to toxic fumes from the pools of waste that lie beneath them. Because they are unable to peck and forage for food, chickens will begin to peck at one another. In order to prevent this, their beaks are seared off, which is not only painful and stressful, but also makes it difficult for the bird to feed normally. During this intense de-beaking process, a number of hens die of shock. Even though there have been countless investigations of egg farms conducted by animal rights groups in the United States, the same things are seen: dead hens in cages with live ones, birds who have lost their feathers from stress, birds suffering from broken bones, bloody open wounds with untreated infection, and blatant physical abuse of these beautiful birds by farm workers. In the United States alone, more than 300 million laying hens produce eggs for human consumption.

Health problems have been found to arise in humans when they eat the flesh or byproducts from these stressed and sickly animals. Unnatural factory-farming conditions create an onslaught of health problems for the animals, such as spawning strains of resistant bacteria like *E. coli and salmonella,* which creates the need for drugs such as antibiotics and hormones. A report from the National Research Council has acknowledged that there is a link between the use of antibiotics in food animals, the development of bacterial resistance to these drugs and human diseases. Antibiotic-resistant bacteria inevitably develop in the cattle, which can easily be transmitted to humans through the consumption of meat or through human contact with living animals. This leads to a reduction in the efficiency of antibiotics in fighting infections and reduced levels of favorable intestinal bacteria, which could increase susceptibility to intestinal infections, such as acute gastroenteritis with fever, pain and diarrhea. A depressed immune system also results, which could lower resistance to infections and increase allergic reactions. Those at the greatest risk include infants, the elderly and those with weakened immune systems.

Factory-farmed processed meat If you want to really understand just what you're eating when you bite into a bologna sandwich or a hot dog, set aside a day and take a field trip through a meat-packing house. It will evoke a multitude of emotions. Not only that, most deli meats contain sodium nitrites and nitrates. Sodium nitrites help to prevent the growth of *Clostridium botulinum,* which can cause botulism in humans and is also used alone or in conjunction with sodium nitrate as a color fixative in cured meat and poultry products, such as bologna, hot dogs and bacon. During the high-heat cooking process, nitrites combine with amines naturally present in meat to form carcinogenic compounds. These carcinogenic compounds have been associated with cancer of the mouth, bladder, esophagus, stomach and brain. Research in Sweden found that Swedes who ate on average 3 ounces of processed meat each day had a 15 percent greater chance of developing stomach cancer than those who consumed 2 ounces or less. The Cancer Research Center of Hawaii and the University of Southern California reported in the *Journal of the National Cancer Institute* (2005; 97:1458-65) that they studied 190,000 people, ages 45 to 75, for seven years. Those who ate the most processed meat, such as bacon, ham and cold cuts, had a 68% higher risk of pancreatic cancer than those who ate the least. "Most" was defined as at least 0.6 ounce processed meat, 1-ounce beef or 0.3-ounce pork per 1,000 calories consumed.

Pasteurized dairy products According to William Campbell Douglass II, M.D. in *The Douglass Report* (2008), a myriad of health problems such as allergies, constipation, arthritis, cancer, and osteoporosis manifest in some form or degree in those who consume processed dairy products. He also states that pasteurized dairy may even diminish our resistance to disease, especially in the young. To make matters worse, pasteurized milk often comes from factory-farmed cows that are typically crammed together and fed not just grains to fatten them up, but also poultry litter from poultry factory farms and ground-up animal parts. These cows are also given hormones to produce more milk faster, and low doses of antibiotics to prevent illness…all of which find their way into the milk you drink. The common practice of pasteurization (the use of high heat to destroy objectionable organisms) also destroys enzymes, which inactivates the effects of these vitally important living elements. One of those living elements is lipase, an enzyme that breaks down fat into amino acids. As a result of destroying the lipase enzyme, a person may become lactose intolerant when drinking pasteurized milk, but not lactose intolerant when drinking unpasteurized milk.

Farm-raised fish While some believe that eating farm-raised fish is a healthy choice, think again. Farm-raised fish, like factory-farmed animals, are often crammed into water tanks next to one another. Diseases proliferate in the feces-tainted waters in which they live. To combat this, these fish are often fed antibiotics. A study published in *Science Magazine* reports that farm-raised salmon is so contaminated with cancer-causing chemicals, including the previously mentioned PCBs, that people should eat it no more than once a month. Of the 14 chemicals studied, most of them pesticides, all are banned in the United States. However, much of the farm-raised fish in your grocery store is grown offshore and not regulated at all by the U.S. FDA when they are shipped into the U.S. These chemicals can linger for decades in the environment and in the human body, and are present in the smaller fish that are ground up and fed to salmon and other large fish raised in giant ocean cages.

Fish are often contaminated by toxic emissions in the form of heavy metals, which are produced by coal-fired power plants, incinerators, and other industrial facilities. This stench ends up in the water and accumulates in fish, especially in those that are higher up the food chain. Ken Cook, president of the Environmental Working Group, reports that some 40 tons of mercury are released into our environment every year by these various industries. Although large fish like tuna, sea bass, marlin, and halibut show some of the worst contamination, dozens of other species and thousands of various other sea forms also show signs of serious pollution. He also reports that as a result of the heavy metal contamination in seafood, women who eat a lot of fish during pregnancy, or even as little as a single serving of a highly contaminated fish, can expose their developing child to excessive levels of mercury. This toxic metal can cross the placental barrier to harm the rapidly developing nervous system, including the brain. Fish such as shrimp, crab, and scallops are reported to have low-mercury levels, but are still ranked in the strong acid-forming food category.

> **Note** For those of you who still want to include fish in your diet, consider fish that are ranked low in toxic chemicals such as mercury. These fish are: salmon, herring, halibut, cod, pike, sardines, tilapia, tuna, mahi mahi, flounder, snapper, whitefish, bluegill sunfish, and lake trout.

Nuts Peanuts are extremely acid-forming and should be eliminated from your diet. I have found that even a small handful of either can turn your next morning urine acid, no matter how many alkalizing foods you've consumed.

Drinks It is estimated that the average American drinks more than 53 gallons of carbonated soft drinks each year. This is more than any other beverage, including milk, beer, coffee, or water. Soft drinks are, unfortunately, amongst the most acid-forming drinks we can consume. This is primarily because carbon dioxide is added to make them fizz, and carbon dioxide added to water produces carbonic acid. The pH of these beverages varies with the amount of carbon dioxide and other ingredients in them, but it is generally extremely acidic, having a pH below 4. Sports and so-called energy drinks are popular with some health-conscious folks. We have been sold on the idea that these drinks hydrate us better than water and are better for us than soft drinks. Unfortunately, this is not true!

Dental researchers are warning us that sports and energy drinks are much worse than soft drinks. Dr. Anthony von Fraunhofer, professor of Biomaterials Science at the University of Maryland Dental School in Baltimore, reported that "enamel damage caused by non-cola and sports beverages was 3-11 times greater than cola-based drinks, with energy drinks and bottled lemonades causing the most harm to dental enamel." Dr. Fraunhofer said that, contrary to popular belief, carbonation per se does not cause cavities but rather, it is the acidity of drinks that causes most of the problems as acids alter the pH level in the mouth. Human saliva, for example, should have a pH level of 6.5 to 7.5. When the pH level falls below 5.5, the bacteria that cause cavities proliferate. He reports, "most soft drinks, from Snapple to Coca-Cola, also contain food additives such as phosphoric acid, citric acid, malic acid and tartaric acid. All of these acids lower the pH level, causing tooth enamel to break down."

To conduct the study, published in the 2005 edition of the *Medical Journal of General Dentistry,* researchers soaked teeth in various popular drinks for a period of 14 hours, an exposure period equivalent to about 13 years' worth of normal beverage consumption. They found the drinks that caused the most enamel to dissolve included KMX sports drink, Snapple lemonade, Red Bull, Lemon-lime Gatorade, PowerAde Arctic Shatter, Arizona Iced Tea, Fanta Orange, and finally Pepsi and Coca-Cola.

Product	Acid	Sugar (12 oz.)
Barq's	4.61	10.7 tsp.
Diet Coke	3.39	0.0
Mountain Dew	3.22	11.0 tsp.
Gatorade	2.95	3.3 tsp
Coke Classic	2.63	9.3 tsp.
Pepsi	2.49	9.8 tsp.
Sprite	3.42	9.0 tsp.
Diet 7-Up	3.67	0.0

Diet Dr. Pepper	3.41	0.0
Surge	3.02	10.0
Gatorade	2.95	3.3
Hawaiian Fruit Punch	2.82	10.2
Orange Minute Maid	2.80	11.2
Dr. Pepper	2.92	9.5
BATTERY ACID	1.00	0.0

The threshold pH for enamel dissolution is 5.5.

Heavy consumers of soft drinks (with or without sugar) excrete huge amounts of calcium, magnesium and other trace minerals into their urine. The more mineral loss, the greater the risk for osteoporosis, osteoarthritis, hypothyroidism, coronary artery disease, high blood pressure, and a long list of degenerative diseases generally associated with premature aging.

Carson E. Pierce of the Alkalize for Health organization reports that one soft drink can cause a sudden change of saliva pH to around 5.5. He says that it takes around 35 glasses of alkaline water, water with a pH of around 10, to neutralize the acid of just one cola or soft drink.

Plastic bottled water While most of us realize the acidifying effects of drinking tap water, most aren't aware of the acidifying effects of drinking water out of plastic bottles. It is estimated that Americans are buying 28 billion petroleum-based plastic water bottles every year in which 8 out of every 10 end up in a landfill. Not only does it take about 1,000 years for those bottles to break down, the process of manufacturing bottled water created more than 2.5 million tons of carbon dioxide, which inevitably ends us acidifying our outer as well as our inner environment. In 2006, it took more than 17 million barrels of oil (excluding the oil used in transporting the plastic) to produce plastic bottles for the bottled water industry.

Researchers have now concluded that certain types of plastic that holds the water have dangerous chemicals, such as phthalates and bisphenol A. They report that these chemicals are seeping into the water, especially when the bottle is left in a hot car, transportation truck, or left in storage crates out in the hot sun too long. These toxins have been found to disrupt the endocrine system, cause fatigue, weight gain and hormone imbalances.

You can avoid a toxin overdose by checking the resin code on the bottom of the bottle. This code tells you what type of plastic it is. Here is a quick rundown on the most commonly used and safest type of plastics.

PET (or PETE) 1: Polyethylene terephthalate, is the type of plastic that is most likely what your clear single-serve water bottle is made of. It has been deemed safe for one-time use, but refilling may increase risk of chemicals leaching out into the water. Not recommended to leave in the hot sun or for re-use.

HDPE 2: High-density polyethylene is a type of plastic that is commonly used for gallon jugs, and has not been linked to any leaching.

PP5: Polypropylene is a plastic that is easily molded. Meaning it is made with fewer chemicals than other plastics, and has not been linked to leaching.

Plastics to avoid:

- #3 polyvinyl Chloride (PVC), it has endocrine disruptors and probable human carcinogens.

- #6 polystyrene (PS) can leach styrene into food and water.

- #7 polycarbonate contains a bisphenol-A (a hormone disruptor). However, it is used in most baby bottles, five-gallon water jugs and reusable sports bottles.

The best way, however, to drink bottled water is to buy it in glass containers. Even still, most bottled waters I have tested with pH drops are acid, with the exception of spring water. Just make sure the spring water you're drinking comes from unpolluted springs.

MILD ACID-FORMING FOODS & DRINKS
(eat in moderation)

Organic grains, legumes, nuts, seeds, berries, and drinks

The foods listed in this section should be organically or biodynamically grown. This is because commercially-grown produce is produced by a corporate agribusiness that promotes and perpetuates the concept of "Better Living Through Chemistry"—a profit-driven industry that has little if any concern about the ecology of the earth or the ecology of the human body. Not only do the fertilizers and pesticides they use acidify and destroy the waters of our earth, they also acidify and destroy the waters of our bodies. And while the "ash" of commercially-grown produce is alkaline in nature to the human body, over time, the toxic chemical residue that remains on or penetrates into this produce can accumulate within our internal environment. Some sources believe that the use of pesticides outweighs any potential health risks, but research suggests otherwise.

According to research on health disorders compiled August 1998 by Richard Pessinger, M.Ed., and Wayne Sinclair, M.D., petroleum-based chemicals and pesticides are found to cause significant weakening effects to the nervous system and immune system after prolonged exposure. Illnesses identified in the medical research include adult and child cancers, numerous neurological disorders, immune system weakening, autoimmune disorders, asthma, allergies, infertility, miscarriage, and child behavior disorders including learning disabilities, mental retardation, hyperactivity and attention deficit disorders (ADD). This is indeed a sign of chronic acidosis.

Their research revealed that petroleum-based pesticides are believed to cause these problems by a variety of routes including—impairing proper DNA (gene) expression, weakening DNA repair, accelerating gene loss, degeneration of the body's detoxification defenses (liver and kidneys) as well as gradual weakening of the brain's primary defense—the blood brain barrier. Identifying a specific chemical as the original cause of these health disorders is difficult and often overlooked, as it typically requires years of exposure for the body's inherent defenses to weaken sufficiently to result in observable health problems. Also, many petroleum chemicals appear to work in tandem to combine their harmful effects making specific identification even more difficult. However, once a chemically induced illness presents itself, a decline in health status appears to continue rapidly as long as exposure continues.

The following fruits and vegetables have been found to be the most contaminated with pesticides when commercially grown. If it's difficult to find organic produce where you live or the increase in price doesn't fit your budget right now, be sure to buy these foods organically or biodynamically grown.

✓ Apples
✓ Bell Peppers
✓ Celery
✓ Cherries
✓ Grapes (imported)
✓ Nectarines

✓ Peaches
✓ Pears
✓ Potatoes
✓ Red Raspberries
✓ Spinach
✓ Strawberries

The following fruits and vegetables have been found to be the least contaminated with pesticides when commercially grown.

✓ Asparagus
✓ Avocados
✓ Bananas
✓ Broccoli
✓ Cauliflower
✓ Corn (sweet)

✓ Kiwi
✓ Mangoes
✓ Onions
✓ Papaya
✓ Pineapples
✓ Sweet Peas

A healthful solution to pesticide overload...

Although most of us wash our strawberries and cherries before eating, studies at the University of Stirling in the United Kingdom show that peel-and-eat fruit such as bananas, oranges, tangerines and cantaloupe are also coated with fat-trapping toxins. "When you peel these foods, toxins can be transferred to the fruit's flesh and subsequently ingested," says Paula Baillie-Hamilton, M.D., Ph.D., environmental-health specialist and author of *Toxic Overload* (Avery, 2005). "But simply washing with dish soap and rinsing before peeling can quickly remove up to 91% of toxins." When washing, just be sure to use a *Go Green* earth-friendly soap.

Organic, on the other hand, is a natural term used for foods that have been grown without the use of synthetic chemicals, especially fertilizers and pesticides. Biodynamic is a term used for foods grown biologically. The difference is this: organic farmers seek to nourish the living component of the soil—the microbial inhabitants that release, transform and transfer nutrients—whereas biodynamic farmers treat the soil as a living organism within its own ecosystem. Biodynamic is the oldest form of organic farming.

Created by Austrian inventor and anthroposophist Rudolf Steiner, biodynamic growing goes further in its approach to organic growing. It uses what some would call unorthodox methodologies to create the most nutritious foods possible. These methods incorporate planetary and cosmic rhythms (different phases of the sun, moon, planets, and stars) to contribute to the life, growth and form of the plant. By paying close attention to a detailed planting calendar, biodynamic farmers are given precise dates and times for everything from the best time to apply homeopathic field sprays and the use of herbal compost preparations to optimum dates and hours for sowing. It also uses crop rotation and companion planting. Crop rotation is the sequential planting of crops which most benefits the soil, and companion planting is a plant association of two or more plant species in close proximity in order that cultural benefits can be derived, such as pest control, higher yields and better conservation of the soil.

One of the biggest consumer complaints in purchasing organic or biodynamic produce is that it generally costs more than conventional produce, and if you're on a budget it can be discouraging.

However, consider this: *a new study shows the superior nutritional value of buying organically-grown produce in comparison to conventionally-grown produce.*

While there has been a long-standing debate over whether organically-grown food is more nutritious than conventionally-grown food, according to the results from a four-year $25 million European-Union funded study, organic food is healthier than conventional produce and may be better at preventing cancer and heart disease. This study was the biggest study of its kind. In a finding that challenges official advice, researchers have shown that fruits and vegetables contain up to 40% more nutrients if they are grown without chemical fertilizers and pesticides. Organic produce also had higher levels of iron and zinc, which are vital nutrients lacking in many people's diets. The findings come from an expert in organic food whose four-year Newcastle University study was funded by the European Union and food companies.

Just keep this in mind when you're at the check-out line: you may be paying a little more for that one biodynamic or organically-grown tomato, but it may also take 3-4 conventionally-grown tomatoes to match up with that one tomato's nutritional value. And ultimately, it's the alkalizing minerals and nutrition in your produce that you're paying and looking for.

Grains & legumes According to Neal Barnard, M.D., New York Times best-selling author and president of the Physicians Committee for Responsible Medicine in Washington, D.C., grains and legumes set the foundation for a healthy plant-based vegetarian diet. Recent media reports have emphasized the health benefits of whole grains and legumes, reporting that fiber and other substances such as antioxidants, lignans, phenolic acids, phytoestrogens and other phytochemicals may help reduce the risk of heart disease, cancer and other chronic diseases. Researchers have concluded that a relationship between wholegrain intake and coronary heart disease is seen with at least a 20% and perhaps a 40% reduction in risk for those who eat wholegrain foods habitually versus those who eat them rarely.

And while grains and beans are healthful and needed by the human body, they tend to be mildly acid-forming due to the fact that they contain phytic acid, also known as phytates. Phytates are phosphorous compounds that bind with minerals such as iron, calcium and zinc, which interferes with their absorption in the body. They also contain enzyme inhibitors that can interfere with digestion. The key to making them healthful versus harmful (more alkaline versus acid) is to soak them in water for 24-36 hours before cooking, sprouting and eating. This process neutralizes the phytates and enzyme inhibitors and assists in pre-digesting them so that all of their nutrients are more available. Proper preparation also helps break down complex sugars, which assists greatly in digestibility.

> *Note* When purchasing grains and legumes, always choose organic. Most commercially-grown grains and legumes come from hybrid seeds.

Soy products Over the years, soy has received a lot of bad press in various health circles. According to the Weston A. Price Foundation in Washington, D.C., many adverse effects of soy consumption are reported in scientific literature, including thyroid disorders, asthma, digestive disorders, calcium deficiencies leading to rickets, high manganese levels leading to brain damage, and endocrine disruption. They report that high levels of phytic acid (phytates) in soy reduce assimilation of calcium, magnesium, copper, iron and zinc. While research is still being conducted about the overall health dangers versus the benefits of soy, there are epidemiological studies showing that soy consumption is associated with lower rates of heart disease and cancer. John Robbins reports in his book, *The Food Revolution,* every possible reason why most of negative accusations regarding soy foods are false. And while soy, in the end, may be found to be a highly beneficial food, there are clear indications are soy's isoflavones should never exceed 25 milligrams (the FDA's maximum safe amount) in any one day.

I have concluded that the more healthful soy food choices are fermented, predigested soy products like miso and tempeh that have been cultured for over a year. Just make sure you are using soybean products that originate with organic soybeans, since most of the North American soy crop is genetically modified (GMO) and treated with toxic chemicals.

Nuts & seeds Nuts and seeds are fatty foods, which are typically the best sources of vitamin E, an immune-enhancing antioxidant and nerve protector. They contain the largest quantity of fat of all unprocessed foods, much of it in the form of essential fatty acids. Vitamins, minerals, amino acids, and carbohydrates are just a part of their remarkable properties. Viewed in their totality, most health advocates agree that nuts and seeds are the "spark of life, a living and perfect food." Like grains and legumes, nuts contain phytates, so they are best consumed after soaking for 24 hours and eaten in small amounts.

Berries Be aware that all acids are not the same. While there are certain acids, such as ellagic acid in fruits like blueberries, that make these fruits acid-forming, these superfoods were designed by nature to inoculate and protect us during specific growing seasons (June-September) from certain strains and viruses that appear during fall and winter. A recent study found that a plant phytochemical found in blueberries strongly inhibited the replication of the influenza virus in cell cultures. While these plants are acid in nature, they are amongst nature's most powerful superfoods and are known to counteract heart disease, cancers, and other types of illnesses. Just remember that they are given to us by nature during a particular season; they were not designed to be eaten year-round. Fruits such as cranberries have been found to reduce the risk of heart disease. Most recently, a study presented at the annual congress of the International Union of Physiological Sciences in March/ April 2005 found that pigs with atherosclerosis (a primary cause of heart disease) that received a daily dose of cranberry powder had restored blood vessel health. Other studies have also found that people who drink unsweetened cranberry juice have higher levels of good (HDL) cholesterol and improved blood vessel function. And, just like blueberries, these fruits are best eaten during their growing season.

Coffee, beer & wine While I'm not encouraging you to drink coffee, beer and wine, I'm reporting that the pH of coffee tends to vary between 5.0-6.9. This variance depends on the blend of the coffee, where the beans come from, and if it was organically or commercially grown. Soils from different regions are also going to have different effect on ph levels. The same also holds true with beer and wine. The acceptable pH range of barrel-conditioned beer is 3.7-4.1. Wines generally have a pH range of 4.5-5.5. Red wine holds a 5-star choice over white wine because it contains more health promoting polyphenols. So, if you're going to consume coffee or any of these alcoholic beverages, be sure to choose wisely. Drink wine without commercially-added sulfites produced by organic or biodynamic vineyards.

START ALKALIZING!
ALKALINE-FORMING FOODS & DRINKS

The foods listed below and in the Alkaline Food Chart at the end of this chapter are among those on the alkaline food chain. Some are more alkalizing than others. The foods listed in the *strong alkaline-forming food* category are highly alkalizing and should be at least 40% of your daily diet. The foods listed in the *mild alkaline-forming food* category are slightly alkalizing and should also be 40% of your diet, totaling 80% of your daily diet.

STRONG ALKALINE-FORMING FOODS & DRINKS
Dark green leafy vegetables

Go Green! Dark green leafy vegetables provide a great variety of colors from the bluish-green of kale to the bright kelly-green of spinach. Leafy greens run the whole gamut of flavors, from sweet to bitter, from peppery to earthy. Great in salads or in a stir-fry, leafy greens provide a whole range of important nutrients and phytochemicals to keep us alkaline and healthy. Green veggies contain a variety of powerful antioxidants that offer cancer-protective properties. In a Swedish study, it was reported that eating three or more servings a week of green leafy vegetables significantly reduced the risk of stomach cancer, the fourth most common cancer in the world. Broccoli sprouts have been reported to contain 10 times or more *sulforaphane,* a cancer-protective substance, than does mature broccoli. Green leafy vegetables have also been shown to significantly decrease the risk of breast cancer and skin cancer.

One of the greatest components of leafy greens is that they contain high levels of chlorophyll. Chlorophyll is the green pigment found in plants and algae and is responsible for capturing the light energy needed for photosynthesis. Green plants, like water, make life on planet Earth possible. The oxygen we breathe comes primarily from the chlorophyll in green plants and, when we ingest lots of chlorophyll-rich plants, they oxygenate our "inner planet" as well. *The higher our oxygen levels, the higher our vitality and the greater our immunity.*

A mystery to ponder about chlorophyll is that it is identical to

> ### *Go Green!*
> *chlorophyll = green foods =*
> *oxygen = perfect Health (pH)*

human blood with one exception: the major element in chlorophyll is magnesium whereas the major element in blood is iron. Thus, I have concluded that chlorophyll-rich foods are the absolute perfect food for human consumption. Leafy greens and green powders such as barley and wheatgrass rank number one out of all of the alkalizing foods. We just need to consume more of them.

Green drinks   Green juices from greens such as wheatgrass and dandelion, are extremely alkaline-forming. Other green juices from green-leafy vegetables like kale and Swiss chard are also very alkalizing.

Green tea   Extremely high in alkalizing minerals and antioxidants, my favorite green tea is "Living Qi Organic Matcha Green Tea" from Japan. This UDSA and IMO (International Maritime Organization) certified organic tea infuses you with energy while relaxing and alkalizing you at the same time.

Ionized alkaline water   Highly charged ionized water is characterized by groups of small cluster-size molecules that are hydrogen-rich, having the ability to penetrate the cell membrane, enabling nutrients to easily enter and wastes to effortlessly exit. While the source of the water we drink is important, the structure of that water, being hydrogen-poor or hydrogen-rich is the most significant key. The second key is to make sure the water has an abundant amount of minerals that supports the water's pH. Drinking water of 8 or above has proven to be a beneficial factor in a person's health.

MILD ALKALINE-FORMING FOODS & DRINKS
All fruits and vegetables

Fruits & vegetables How many times have you been told, "Eat your veggies?" And how about the cliché, "An apple a day keeps the doctor away?" With all of the latest scientific reports and studies, it seems that both of these clichés are truisms. Eating a diet high in fruits and vegetables is one of the best things you can do for your health. Fruits and vegetables are not only alkalizing, they contain essential vitamins, minerals, fiber and various other phytonutrients that may help protect you from chronic diseases. Compared with people who consume a diet with only small amounts of fruits and vegetables, those who eat generous amounts are likely to have reduced risk of chronic diseases, including stroke, cardiovascular diseases and certain cancers.

According to the United States Department of Agriculture

- Eating a diet rich in fruits and vegetables as part of an overall healthy diet may reduce risk for stroke and perhaps other cardiovascular diseases.

- Eating a diet rich in fruits and vegetables as part of an overall healthy diet may reduce risk for type-2 diabetes.

- Eating a diet rich in fruits and vegetables as part of an overall healthy diet may protect against certain cancers, such as mouth, stomach and colorectal cancer.

- Diets rich in foods containing fiber, such as fruits and vegetables, may reduce the risk of coronary heart disease.

- Eating fruits and vegetables rich in potassium as part of an overall healthy diet may reduce the risk of developing kidney stones and may help to decrease bone loss.

- Eating more foods such as vegetables that are low in calories per cup (instead of higher-calorie foods may help lower calorie intake.

For those of you who have busy lives and believe that a fast-food drive thru is your only grab-and-go option, well you can change that perception right now. Fruits and vegetables are the ultimate fast food. With fruit, all you have to do is peel-and-go, and with vegetables all you have to do is wash-and-go. It's simple and deliciously alkalizing. And best of all, it doesn't cause your 'engine' to go, ping-ping-ping!

Fruit & vegetable juices Freshly-prepared fruit and vegetable juices are powerful way to drink your way to alkaline health. So enjoy as much as you want every day!

Herbal teas Most herbal teas are alkaline-forming; teas such as, chamomile, peppermint, lemon zing or cardamom. These teas are a great tea-time substitute "coffee-break" pleasure.

So what's the solution to both our inner and outer environmental crisis—a crisis that evokes a systemic ecological breakdown? The solution is to stop burning the wrong types of food for fuel into your internal environment. These foods (fuel) cause an internal acid rain, which burns your inner rainforest and depletes your life-giving oxygen. To avoid the impending disasters of global warming, an inflammatory process that occurs because of over-acidification, the answer is to stop acidifying and start alkalizing!

ACID FOOD CHART

STRONG ACID FOODS
(completely eliminate)

Highly Refined Food Items

Salt	Oil	Sugar	Artificial Sweeteners

Highly Processed Junk Foods

Potato Chips	Theatre Popcorn	Roasted Nuts	Fried Hamburgers
Fried Chicken	Fried Fish & Chips	French Fries	Nachos
Cheese Pizza	Breakfast Cereals	White Bread	White Rice
Semolina Pasta	Wheat Bread	Cookies	Cakes
Candy	Puddings	Pies	Ice Cream
Pickles	Pickled Olives	Canned Foods	TV Dinners

Fake Dairy

Cheese Dips	Fake Cheese	Margarine

Processed Fruits

Canned Fruit w/Syrup	Dried Fruits w/Sulfur	Jellies	Jams

Commercial Condiments

Distilled Vinegar	Ketchup	Mustard	Mayonnaise
Relish	Soy Sauce	Salad Dressings	Sauces

Animal Meat

Red Meat	Pork	Chicken	Bison
Veal	Organ Meats	Turkey	Lamb

Wildlife

Duck	Quail	Deer	Rabbit

Pasteurized Dairy Products

Milk	Cream	Cheese	Yogurt
Butter	Sour Cream	Cream Cheese	Cottage Cheese

Processed Meats

Sandwich Meats	Bologna	Spam	Hot Dogs
Ham	Bacon	Sausage	Smoked Meat
Pepperoni	Salami		

Toxic Fish

Farm-Raised Fish	Scallops	Shrimp	Oysters
Crab	Clams	Caviar	Lobster
South Atlantic Grouper	Large Mouth Bass	Perch	Sea Bass
Marlin	King Mackerel	Tilefish	Halibut
Pike	Walleye	White Croaker	Catfish
Shark	Swordfish	Tuna Steaks	Canned Tuna

Less-Toxic Fish

Salmon	Herring	Haddock	Halibut
Cod	Pike	Sardines	Tilapia
Tuna	Mahi Mahi	Flounder	Snapper
Whitefish	Bluegill Sunfish	Lake Trout	

Bottled Beverages

Soft Drinks	Sports Drinks	Plastic Bottled Water

Nuts

Peanut	Cashew	Roasted Nuts

MILD ACID FOODS
(20% of your daily diet)

Organic Grains

Barley	Buckwheat	Basmati Rice	Brown Rice
Wild Rice	Quinoa	Buckwheat	Oat Groats
Wheatberries			

Organic Grain Products

Cornmeal	Popcorn	Corn Nuts	Oatmeal
Sprouted Gread	Rye Bread	Spelt Bread	Hemp Bread
Whole Grain Crackers	Whole Grain Pasta	Whole Grain Pancakes	

Organic Beans

Adzuki Beans	Black Beans	Black-Eyed Peas	Lentils
Chickpeas	Fava Beans	Kidney Beans	Great Northern
Mung Beans	Navy Beans	White Beans	
Pinto Beans	Split Peas	Whole Peas	

Organic Soy Products

Soybeans	Edamame	Tofu	Soymilk
Soy Oil	Soy Baby Formula	Soy Hotdogs	Soy Burgers
Soy Yogurt	Soy Protein (TVP)		

Organic Fermented Soy Products

Miso	Tempeh	Unpasteurized Soy Sauce

Organic Nuts

Acorn	Brazil	Chestnut	Filbert
Hazelnut	Macadamia	Pecan	Walnut

Organic Seeds

Poppy	Sesame	Sunflower	Pumpkin
Hemp	Chia	Flax	

Organic Fruits

Cranberries	Blueberries	Plums	Prunes
Raspberries	Blackberries		

Organic Vegetables

Corn	Winter Squash	White Asparagus Tips

Organic Condiments

Gelatin	Salad Dressings	Vegannaise	Ketchup
Maple Syrup	Raw Honey	Molasses	Mustard
Horseradish	Pickles	Tapioca	Raw Apple Cider
Vinegar			

*Organic Raw Dairy Products

Cow Milk	Goat Milk	Butter	Cow Cheese
Kefir	Yogurt	Cottage Cheese	Goat Cheese

* While organic raw dairy products tend to be only mildly acidic, I am not recommending them as a part of the *Get Clean Go Green EcoDiet Program.*

ALKALINE FOOD CHART

STRONG ALKALINE FOODS
(40% of your daily diet)

Organic Green Leafy Vegetables

Arugula	Beet Greens	Chicory	Collard
Dandelion	Endive	Escarole	Mustard
Kale	Parsley	Sorrel	Spinach
Swiss Chard	Watercress		

Organic Green Powders

Blue Green Algae	Barley Green	Spirulina	Kamut
Alfalfa	Wheatgrass	Green Superfoods	

MILD ALKALINE FOODS
(40% of your daily diet)

Organic Vegetables

Artichokes	Asparagus	Alfalfa Sprouts	Bamboo Shoots
Beets	Broccoli	Brussels Sprouts	Cabbages
Carrots	Celery	Cauliflower	Cucumber
Dill	Sea Vegetables	Eggplant	Garlic
Jerusalem Artichokes	Ginger	Green Beans	Horseradish
Leeks	Lettuce	Mushrooms	Okra
Onions	Parsley	Parsnips	Peas
Peppers	Potatoes	Pumpkin	Radishes
Rutabagas	Sprouts	Squash	Sweet Potatoes
Tomatoes	Turnips	Yams	

Organic Fruits

Apples	Apricots	Avocados	Bananas
Berries (Most)	Cantaloupe	Carob	Cherries
Currants	Dates	Figs	Grapes
Grapefruit	Guavas	Kiwi	Kumquats
Lemons	Limes	Loganberries	Loquats
Mangoes	Nectarines	Olives	Oranges
Papayas	Passion Fruit	Peaches	Pears
Persimmons	Pineapple	Pomegranates	Melons
Dried Fruits	Raspberries	Strawberries	Tamarind

Organic Grains

Amaranth	Millet

Organic Beans

Lima Beans

Organic Miscellaneous Items

Sea Vegetables	Raw Cane Sugar	Raw Honey	Arrowroot
Agar Agar	Kudzu Root	Culinary Herbs	Raw Olives
Blackstrap Molassas	Sauerkraut	Umeboshi Plums	Almond Butter
Sun-Dried Tomatoes	Most Spices	Nutritional Yeast	

Organic Nuts

Almonds	Chestnuts	Coconut	Pine Nuts

Organic Drinks

Unpasteurized Wine	Almond Milk	Hempseed Milk	Coconut Milk
Herbal Teas	Ionized Alkaline Water		

NEUTRAL pH

Organic Oils

Hemp	Olive	Flaxseed	Grapeseed
Sunflower	Pumpkin	Coconut	Udo's Oil Blend
Earth Balance Spread	Sesame		

THE 80/20 ECODIET DAILY MENU

80% Alkaline Foods & Drinks

✓ 40% from the strong alkaline-forming list

✓ 40% from the mild alkaline-forming list

20% Acid Foods & Drinks

✓ 20% from the mild acid-forming list

CHAPTER SEVEN

The Four "Fuel" Groups

Food isn't just something delectable you put in your mouth, chew and swallow. It's any macro or micro substance that provides every cell of your body with the nutrients needed for energy and growth. And while one aspect of achieving a perfect state of health and wellbeing does come from the plant foods picked from organic rich soil, keep in mind that these foods are grown in the earth by the earth with the assistance of air, sunlight and water. As such, your body, your eco-house, also needs to be constantly bathed in these other three elements.

The four elemental forces of air, fire, earth, and water are not only the very elements your body is made of, they are the very dynamics that control the entire physical universe. In fact, they are the basic principles that shaped the first four days of creation and are the basic principles that shaped your body. Therefore, to achieve perfect health, you must align yourself with these principles and fuel your body with the air you breath, the sunlight you absorb, the plants you eat, and the water you drink. These powerful four do not ascend within the structure of a

The original meaning of "eco" comes from the Greek word oikos which means house or habitat; the second meaning is ecological environment.

man-made four food group pyramid, as each are the "pillars" of your house and work together in a synergistic field of movement and are of equal importance.

Because these powerful four create the "pillars" of your house, they are the four "pillars" of the *Get Clean Go Green EcoDiet*. Follow their basic principles of creation and, in turn, you'll create a state of health and wellbeing, not just for yourself but for the planet at large, that far surpasses the scope of most our imaginations.

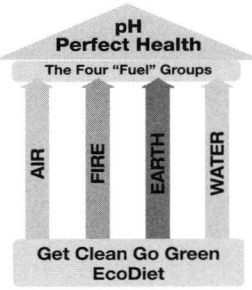

Just remember that no matter what SOS symptoms you may be experiencing or whatever disease name you may have been tagged with, if you work *with* these four powerful forces of nature and not *against* them, you *can* turn your environmental crisis around.

AIR—The Alkaline Breath

Like the wind circulates air throughout our planet's atmosphere, our breath circulates air throughout our body's atmosphere, cleansing, oxygenating and alkalizing every cell of our bodies. Air is our most vital food. Our breath removes acids and alkalizes us like nothing else. With the sheer movement of breathing out carbon dioxide, our blood is actually alkalized. To keep this process working, there must be a constant exchange of oxygen and carbon dioxide.

"Breathing is the FIRST place not the LAST place one should investigate when any disordered energy presents itself."

–Sheldon Saul Hendler, M.D., Ph.D., author of *The Oxygen Breakthrough*

In fact, there is no other modality by which our blood turns acid or alkaline than breathing. But we have forgotten how to breathe properly.

We have become a nation of stress-driven, sedentary-shallow chest breathers. Most of us are taking a minimal amount of breath into our lungs, generally by drawing air into the chest area using the intercostals muscle instead of through the lungs via our diaphragm. Most chest breathers breathe shallowly throughout the day and are almost always unaware of it. Shallow breathing causes a build up of carbon dioxide in the blood, which causes the blood to become acidic. Many of our health problems, which generally goes undiagnosed, can often be traced back to shallow breathing. But when we learn how to breathe correctly, our breath can have a powerful influence on our overall health.

> *"If I had to limit my advice on healthier living to just one tip, it would be simply to learn how to breathe correctly."*
>
> – Andrew Weil, M.D., author of *Eight Weeks to Optimal Health*

The diaphragm is a dome-shaped structure that acts as a natural partition between our heart and lungs and organs. When we take a full deep breathe, the diaphragm moves through its entire range downward to massage and oxygenate the liver, stomach, and other organs and tissues below it, and upward to massage and oxygenate the heart. Also, with a full deep breathe, the diaphragm moves farther down into the abdomen, assisting our lungs to expand more completely into the chest cavity.

This means that, with each breath, more oxygen is taken in and more carbon dioxide is eliminated. It also means that with each full, deep breath, we're increasing blood flow and peristalsis and pumping the lymph more efficiently throughout our lymphatic system. The lymphatic system, which is an important part of our immune system, has no other means of pumping the lymph other than muscular movements, including the movements of breathing.

Consider this:

- Science has proven that cancer is anaerobic, it does not survive in high levels of oxygen.

- Shortness of breath and heart disease are directly linked - the heart goes into spasm when it is deprived of oxygen.

- Studies have shown that there is a high correlation between high blood pressure and poor breathing.

- Most emotional issues, including anxiety and depression, result from the nervous system being out of balance. Breathing drives the nervous system.

- Optimal breathing helps to promote weight loss. Oxygen burns fat and calories. Breathing well is the key to sleeping well and waking up feeling rested. Breathing provides 99% of your energy. Without energy, nothing works.

- Virtually every health condition and human activity is improved with optimal breathing.

- Clinical studies prove that oxygen, wellness, and life-span are totally dependent on proper breathing. Lung volume is a primary marker for how long you will live.

The most pervasive reason we have forgotten how to breath properly is that we have been strongly impacted by our sedentary modern-day society. Movement causes us to breathe and our breath is the fuel that will create that healthier, happier *you* that you were designed to be.

Breathing Practices

Learning to develop the power of your breath is of the utmost importance. It is an indispensable aid to superior health, peak performance, and life extension. Let's try a few.

(1) Sit comfortably with eyes open or shut. With mouth closed, inhale and exhale several times. Next, begin slowly exhaling through your nose, counting to seven, starting at the top of your chest, moving down through your mid-torso and into your diaphragm. Pause for seven counts. Begin inhaling slowly through your nose, counting to seven, starting at your diaphragm, expanding your belly, then your mid-torso, and lastly the top of your chest. Pause for seven counts and exhale as before. Repeat 5-10 times.

(2) Once again, sit in a comfortable position. With mouth closed, breathe in and out through your nose as fast and equally as possible. Continue for 10-15 seconds at first, and then as you become more accustomed to this type of rapid

breath, increase it to one full minute. This breath practice is a very ancient belly breath that energizes you while toning the abdomen and massaging the internal organs and lymph system. This type of breathing activates the lungs, neck, chest and abdomen.

Breathe Deeply & Slim Down

If you find it's tough to exercise on a regular basis, try deep breathing exercises, which can be done anytime, anywhere. Deep breathing greatly assists in facilitating weight loss due to the fact that large amounts of oxygen causes the chemical reactions in your body to take place much faster, thus you burn more calories than you take in.

This in turn speeds up your metabolism and makes you burn more body fat. Body fat is also eliminated with the release of carbon dioxide. In a relatively short time you'll not only feel the difference, you'll see the difference. The answer is to simply breathe deeply and do it often throughout the day.

Always remember, whenever you feel stressed, *breathe!* If stress isn't managed properly, your body will burn glycogen, not fat, for that extra energy needed. Just by triggering a relaxation response by using a few deep breaths, your body is encouraged to burn fat instead.

> *"Lack of activity destroys the good condition of every human being, while movement and methodical physical exercise save it and preserve it."*
>
> – Plato, Greek philosopher and Mathematician

The following deep breathing exercises can be performed sitting down or standing up. Let's try a few.

(1) Begin by blowing all of the air out of your lungs through your mouth. When you feel as though you don't have any more air to expel, give it one more thrust, completely emptying your lungs. Relax for a few seconds. Close your mouth and quickly inhale through your nose, pulling as much air into your lungs as possible, always focusing your breath onto the area of the diaphragm

(the diaphragm is located just below the sternum in the "V" formed by the rib cage). As the diaphragm expands, the lower abdomen should rise slightly, followed by the chest (note that if you're not making a noise, you're most likely not doing it right). Continue to steadily pull the air in as deeply as you can, completely filling your lungs.

When you feel as if you've taken in all the air you can, open your mouth and take a final gasp of air in through your mouth. Hold for 7-10 seconds. Open your mouth wide and exhale from the diaphragm with a quick, explosive breath through your mouth. Again, you should breathe out hard enough that you are able to hear the noise as you force the air from deep inside. Continue exhaling, completely emptying your lungs. As you blow the air out, roll your stomach in and up. This is the most important step, particularly if you want to flatten your stomach, tone your abdominal muscles and oxygenate every cell of your body.

(2) My favorite deep-breathing exercise is rebounding on a mini-trampoline. And, it's easy to fit it into your daily routine. I often rebound several times a day while watching Oprah or listening to music. Some scientists have even concluded that jumping on a mini-trampoline is one of the most effective exercises yet devised by man, especially because of the effect rebounding has on the lymph system.

The lymph fluid moves through channels called "vessels" that are filled with one way valves, so the lymph always moves in the same direction. The main lymph vessels run up the legs, up the arms and up the torso. This is why the vertical up and down movement of rebounding is so effective to pump the lymph.

The mini-trampoline subjects the body to gravitational pulls ranging from zero at the top of each bounce to 2-3 times the force of gravity at the bottom, depending on how high a person is rebounding. This gravitation pull pumps the lymph like nothing else. Then, when you add deep-breathing exercises to your rebounding bounce, the alkalizing effect goes off the chart!

Just be sure to consume lots of organic fruit, green leafy vegetables and sprouts. This is because your body needs adequate amounts of high quality glucose to maintain high oxygen levels as the whole purpose of oxygen is to combine with glucose to manufacture ATP (adenosine triphosphate) in the cells, which powers the whole process of life. Most people who tend to be shallow breathers are low in high-quality glucose because the extra oxygen simply cannot be used. This is why the *EcoDiet* consists of 80% fruits and green-leafy vegetables.

Indoor Air Pollution

Before taking your next deep breath, you may want to consider the quality of the indoor air you're breathing. According to an EPA report to Congress on Indoor Air and the subcommittee hearings on the Indoor Air Quality Act of 1989, indoor air pollution is one of the nation's most important environmental health concerns. At the turn of the 21st century, it was estimated that the average household contained more chemicals than found in a typical chemistry laboratory.

> *"Of chemicals commonly found in homes, 150 have been linked to allergies, birth defects, cancer and psychological abnormalities."*
>
> – Consumer Product Safety Commission

It has also been estimated that most homes have airborne concentrations of hazardous and toxic chemicals that are two to five times higher indoors than outdoors. In one five-year study, the EPA reported that a number of homes had chemical levels that were seventy times higher inside the home than outside the home.

In a study conducted over a fifteen-year period, it was found that women who worked at home had a 54% higher death rate from cancer than women who had jobs away from home. The study concluded that the increased death rate in women is mostly due to the daily exposure of hazardous chemicals found in ordinary household products.

The studies also revealed the following:

- Toxic chemicals in household cleaners are three times more likely to cause cancer than outdoor air pollution.

- Women who are exposed to solvents experience a higher than normal rate of spontaneous abortion.

- Studies of umbilical cords of newborns revealed the presence of approximately 100 synthetic chemicals.

- Heart palpitations, insomnia, night sweats and hormonal imbalances are signs of chemical poisoning.

- People prone to headaches and slight disorientation may find environmental chemical toxicity to be the cause.

- Toxic chemical fumes can cause excessive fatigue and trigger unexplained flu-like symptoms.

- Dioxin exposure is linked to cancer and is considered a possible cause of endometriosis.

- Exposure to certain chemicals is known to contribute to the development of heart disease.

- Impaired memory and concentration, auditory and visual perception is linked to excessive exposure to toxic chemicals.

The EPA reports that most household and personal care products release toxic vapors into the air when they are used, and even when they are stored. This process is called outgassing, the slow release of a gas that was once trapped in some type of material. It is important to note that outgassing is exacerbated when windows are sealed and fresh air from the outside is not permitted in, thus, only re-circulated air from heaters and air conditioning systems are breathed by inhabitants.

The next and most important consideration with regards to outgassing is our children. Consider the following:

- Children spend between twelve and twenty-two hours a day indoors.

- Children are physiologically more vulnerable to toxic vapors than adults because of their higher metabolic rate.

- Children require more oxygen than adults, they breathe in two to three times as much air (and therefore toxins) relative to body size than adults.

- Children are more physically active, which increases their breathing rate and intake of toxins.

- Children generally play close to the floor where heavier pollutants settle.

Airborne household chemicals are also a suspected cause of Sudden Infant Death Syndrome (SIDS), which takes the lives of thousands of infants each year. This may explain the documented higher incidence of SIDS in the wintertime. This, of course, is because windows are left closed, which decreases ventilation and increases the concentration of outgassed vapors.

To circumvent possible outgassing in your home, read every label on your various cleaners, laundry supplies, hairsprays, make-up, shampoos, soaps, crèmes, dishwashing detergents, shoe and furniture polishes, insect repellants, etc., that sits on your shelves. If they are not eco-friendly biodegradable products, the ingredients most likely consists of the following:

Formaldehyde is a toxic gas that is used in many every day personal care and household cleaning products, such as nail polish, glue and adhesives, disinfectants, cosmetics, shampoos, hair conditioners, air fresheners, household antiseptics, carpet cleaners, mouth washes, etc., a list that can be unending. This toxic chemical has been associated with blood-cell abnormalities that are characteristic of leukemia, a cancer of the blood or bone marrow.

Dioxin is a dangerous chemical found in every day household products like chlorine bleach. Once outgassed in the environment, this chemicals accumulates in both people and animals. Hundreds of studies have shown a direct link between dioxin exposure and cancer, birth defects, and developmental and reproductive disorders.

Ammonia is toxic when inhaled in concentrated vapors and is considered hazardous waste. Ammonia is found in all-purpose cleansers, glass cleaners, laundry detergents and metal polishers.

Chlorinated cleaners can be especially toxic. Some cleaners contain dioxin, a known carcinogen that can build up in the food chain, is stored in fat cells and is believed to affect the endocrine system. Chlorinated materials are used in bleach, dishwasher detergents and toilet bowl cleaners.

Glycol ether is a central nervous system depressant that can poison the kidney and liver. It is often found in all-purpose cleaners and some laundry detergents.

Lye or Sodium Hydroxide is in most oven cleaners and is a corrosive poison and hazardous waste.

Oxalic acid is caustic and corrosive to skin and mucous membranes. It is commonly added to cleanser, toilet bowl cleaners and metal polishes.

Petroleum-based detergents contain neurotoxins and central nervous system depressants. Exotic sounding chemicals like nonyl phenol and alkyl phenol ethoxylates (APEs) are found in detergents, furniture polish, cosmetics and household cleaners, and contain environmental impurities that contribute to pollution.

Phosphates are added to dishwashing and laundry detergents because they act as a water softener. Phosphates are released into the environment through wastewater and are not removed by sewage treatment systems. Phosphates can cause algae overgrowth and suffocation of aquatic life.

The Top 12 Killers:

- Bug Killers
- Mold & Mildew Cleaners
- Oven Cleaners
- Dishwasher Detergent
- Car Care Products
- Laundry Products
- All Purpose Cleaners
- Carpet Shampoo
- Ammonia
- Drain Cleaner
- Furniture Polish
- Bleach

Fortunately, there are three ways to reduce your family's exposure to hazardous airborne toxins from household products: (1) eliminate every chemically-laden household cleaning and personal care product that sits on your shelves—this includes laundry detergents, dryer sheets, all-purpose cleaners, dishwashing liquids, shampoo and hair conditioners, hand and body soaps, nail polish and nail polish remover, (2) use non-toxic, ecofriendly products…products that can be purchased from various distributors or from your local health food store and (3) purify your indoor air by using a reputable, top-notch air purifier.

FIRE—The Alkaline Sun

Today most of us have lost our personal relationship with the sun and its relationship with us. Throughout the history of time, we've gone from worshipping it to shunning it, both in the religious sense as well as in the bronzed sense. While every living thing upon our planet is dependent upon the light of the sun, we've been made to believe that it's our enemy. We think that the sun is something to be shunned and avoided and that sunbathing and sun-gazing are dangerous practices that can destroy our retinas, age our skin and often cause skin cancer. Current scientific research, however, exposes these narrow archaic myths. Let us now reconsider ending our on-again, off-again relationship with sunlight and open to an understanding of its importance towards achieving a state of health and wellbeing.

Eat Light

Michael Holick, M.D., the world's foremost authority on vitamin D and the healing power of natural sunlight, says that adequate amounts of sensible sun exposure during childhood not only maximizes the bone health of children but may even decrease their risk of many chronic diseases in later life including type-1 diabetes, multiple sclerosis, rheumatoid arthritis and common cancers.

In his book, *The UV Advantage,* Dr. Holick states how vitamin D deficiencies can cause prostate cancer, breast cancer, cervical cancer, osteoporosis, rickets and various other diseases. According to two recent studies, he recommends that increasing vitamin D intake through sunlight, diet and/or supplements may decrease a person's risk of contracting breast cancer by 50% and of contracting colorectal cancer by more than 65%. Several studies have shown that exposure to natural sunlight increases the number of white blood cells in the body, which plays the leading role in defending against invasions by bacteria and foreign organisms. Because of the increase in white blood cell activity after sunlight exposure, a person's ability to fight infections is greatly increased along with the body's ability to stop the reproduction of viruses.

While it's important that we absorb the rays of the sun each day, like most anything else, sunbathing can be overdone. The sun must be treated with great respect. The skin must be properly conditioned to sunlight. Too much sun during the wrong time of day is definitely unwise. The best time to get sunlight is before 10am or after 3pm, a time when the UV rays are less potent. Start with 15 minutes either early morning (9am) or late afternoon (4pm). Add 15 more minutes each day until you have a healthy, bronze tan. Remember, the less clothing or covering the better. So, when it comes to properly absorbing the rays of the sun, remember to always *eat light!*

Drink Your Sunscreen

Concern about skin cancer is valid, especially if you're a redhead with light skin. However, most sunscreen products can cause more harm than good. Some sunscreen products contain toxic chemicals that, when they penetrate through the skin, can actually increase the risk of disease. Toxic chemicals you may wish to avoid include: PABA, Dioxybenzone, Oxybenzone, and Titanium Dioxide. Another major problem with sunscreen is that it blocks the skin's ability to produce vitamin D by more than 95%.

The answer may just be as simple as eating or drinking more fresh vegetables and berries, foods that are loaded with phytochemicals, such as antioxidants. Modern nutritional science has recently discovered new insights into how an increase of antioxidants helps to protect our skin naturally. In fact, studies on other phytochemicals, such as polyphenols and nutrients such as vitamin C, have shown that it definitely offers protection from UVA radiation and that nutritional factors exert promising effects on the skin. These are just a few examples:

Foods That Protect You

Red, yellow and orange fruits and veggies
These contain carotenoids, which reduce sunburn.

Tart cherries and peppermint leaves
These contain perilly alcohol, which stops cancer formation in
human cells exposed to intense UV light.

Leafy greens
These contain lutein and zeaxanthin, which stops UV-induced
cell proliferation.

Green tea
This contains antioxidants EGCGs, which block DNA damage in
light-exposed human skin cells.

Oranges, lemons and limes
These contain limonene, which is linked to a 34% reduction in skin cancer.

So, why not drink your sunscreen? Try a cup of warm green tea in the morning
or blend up a delectable fruit smoothie or juice a carotenoid-rich green drink. The
more you drink, the greater your protection.

Sunscreen Smoothie

1 large orange, peeled
12 strawberries, stemmed
1 banana, peeled
1 tablespoon green powder
Blend at high speed until smooth.

Leafy Green Sunscreen

8 stalks celery
4 kale leaves or Swiss chard

1 bunch parsley
1 handful spinach
Juice.

Sun-Gazing Practices

Sun-gazing is a term broadly applied to an ancient practice of staring directly at the sun at sunrise or sunset. This practice takes place during the first or last 30 minutes of the day so that UV radiation is at its minimum. If great caution is used, i.e. staring at the sun for shorter periods of time then gradually working up to longer amounts of time, retina damage to the eyes can be avoided. As an interesting side bar, sun-gazing during a solar eclipse is not recommended.

While there has not been any scientific evidence to substantiate the beneficial claims of sun-gazing, there are reports that suggest gazing is capable of providing the sun-gazer with a sense of physical, mental, emotional, and spiritual wellbeing. Some even report a decrease in irritability, anger and frustration and an increase in memory. Others even claim a complete relief from almost every disease known.

Sun-gazing is often practiced with bare feet in direct contact with the earth. You begin by staring directly at the rising sun for ten seconds then adding an additional ten seconds to the total sun-gazing time each consecutive day until you are staring at the sun for 45 minutes. In six months, some have experienced the feeling of hunger dissipate, and after ten months others claim that they never need to eat again!

In other words, they are *eating light;* sunlight has become the primary food they're burning for energy. It is alleged that after 45 minutes of sun-gazing, one would be full of light energy, just like a solar-charged battery, with no need to continue the sun-gazing practice. Some report that at this point, a person is able to utilize over 50% of their brain. If these claims hold true, the implications could be staggering.

EARTH —The Alkaline Foods

Like planet Earth, the human body is a living organism that is alkaline by design. Thus, to sustain optimal health and foster longevity, we must eat a living foods, plant-based alkaline diet. This means that the foods we burn for fuel must be grown in organic soil, come from seed-bearing plants, and be consumed in their whole, natural, unadulterated state. Various studies have been conducted by the Weston A. Price Foundation on the subject of dietary habits and their relationship to the health and longevity of primitive people and tribal cultures around the globe. Weston A. Price, DDS, traveled worldwide in his search. He discovered that isolated primitives, whose diets consisted of natural, fresh unprocessed foods grown in their own environment, had virtually no dental caries, disease, loss of sight or hearing, gray hair or tooth decay, even when they were eating large quantities of raw sugar cane. On the other hand, those who were subject to dental decay and various other degenerative diseases were found to have modernized their diets, eating denatured, cooked, processed foods such as white bread, white rice and white sugar. He concluded that as long as the foods eaten were natural, unprocessed and mostly raw, the people maintained good health and long lives. Thus, a living foods, plant based alkaline diet is an absolute must for those who are searching for optimal health.

Eat Raw, Living Foods

Having a diet consisting of 75-100% raw foods is called a raw living foods diet. If 75-100% of a person's total food consumption is raw food, they are considered a raw foodist. Raw foodism promotes a lifestyle where the majority of foods eaten are in their natural organic state, foods that are uncooked and unprocessed. The greater the percentage of raw food in the diet, the greater the health benefits. Raw foods are considered living foods because they contain enzymes.

Enzymes are active proteins contained in all living things, whether human or vegetable, making them one of the "keys of life." Enzymes catalyze and regulate nearly every biochemical reaction within all living cells, making them absolutely necessary for feeding and cleansing our cellular structure. The utilization of individual enzymes for specific applications has long been recognized as an effective way to help the human body handle stressful situations. Enzymes are being constantly used up and excreted through sweat and urine. If we don't replace them through proper diet, the body will replace enzymes from within itself, borrowing from metabolic processes causing chronic fatigue, cellular and organ exhaustion, disease and eventually death. This is where food plays a very significant role.

For the most part, foods are composed of proteins, fats, and carbohydrates. The foods we eat are digested in stages being broken down along the way by approximately 22 different digestive enzymes made by the body. For instance, protease breaks down proteins into amino acids, lipase breaks down fats into fatty acids and amylase breaks down carbohydrates into double sugars. Chewing our food well is significant to release these enzymes.

When foods are consumed in their raw natural state, they contain high amounts of enzymes. Enzymes accelerate the flavor, color, texture, and nutritional changes in plant foods, especially when they are cut, sliced, crushed, bruised, and exposed to air. Enzymes are very sensitive to heat above 118°F. Thus, when food is cooked, steamed, canned, pasteurized, baked, or boiled above 120°F, it has lost virtually all enzyme activity. Max Planck Institute actually reports that if you cook your food, you destroy 50-70% of the food's protein, 70-90% of the food's vitamins and phytonutrients, and 100% of the food's enzymes.

Thus, eating a diet high in raw, living foods is the absolute healthiest way to eat, even if the other 25% of your diet consists of various cooked foods such as brown rice or beans. That 25% can even include an occasional organic blueberry muffin or carrot cake.

Living foods include organic vegetables, wheat sprouts, seeds and nuts of every variety, fruits, berries and wild greens. Raw root vegetables, vine vegetables, edible bush berries and tree fruits are some of my favorite living fruits. While a raw food diet is usually equated with raw veganism in which only raw plant foods are eaten, depending on the type of lifestyle and results desired, some raw foodists (and I'm not one of them nor do I advocate it) emphasize raw meat and other raw animal products such as raw milk, eggs and cheese.

Adherents of raw foodism believe that consumption of uncooked foods encourages weight loss and prevents and/or heals many forms of sickness and chronic diseases. In fact, Dr. Gabriel Cousins, M.D., states in his DVD, "Raw for 30 Days," that he has clinically proven that those who consume a 100% raw living foods diet can turn around both type-1 and type-2 diabetes in 30 days.

Let's Get Juiced!

One of the fastest ways to restore your internal environment back into a perfect state of health and wellbeing is to *get juiced!* Drinking an enormous amount of freshly extracted vegetable juices every day is like having a blood transfusion from nature's hospital. In fact, this is what I did 30 years ago when I got sick and was unsure if I was going to live from one day to the next. After reading Dr. Norman Walker's book (who lived to be around 120), *Fresh Vegetable and Fruit Juices,* and understanding that the juice of the plant is the blood of the plant, I put my new juice machine to the test.

For 40 days and 40 nights, I drank 3-4 quarts of various vegetable juice blends every day. After that, I kept drinking the same amount of juice, but I also ate a green leafy salad plus fresh organic fruits in season. I ate no nuts, no seeds, no grains, no beans, and no oils. My family thought I had lost my mind, but what I had truly lost was an immune deficient, disease-ridden body. The superbug that had made my body its home had no more food supply, so it had no other choice but to pack up and leave.

Fresh vegetable and fruit juices provide the body's intelligence (the healer within) with an enormous amount of raw building materials such as vitamins, minerals, phytonutrients, and enzymes it needs in order to restore ecological balance back into your internal terrain. What I discovered is that if you provide the intelligence of your body with the right materials in the right amount, it knows exactly how to restore what has been lost.

So go ahead. For the health of it … *get juiced* … you'll be glad you did!

Enjoy A Daily Smoothie

Science has recently discovered that plants convert solar energy into complex chemical compounds called phytochemicals, also called phytonutrients, contained in plant foods such as fruits, berries, vegetables, whole grains, legumes, nuts, and seeds. When you plant a seed into rich soil, it uses the power of the sun to draw nutrients from the soil to convert inorganic substances into organic substances. In turn, these nutrients power all living organisms on earth. Currently, the terms *phytochemical* and *phytonutrient* are being used interchangeably to describe the biologically active compounds of plants considered to have a highly beneficial effect on human health. These compounds, such as anthocyanins, which are flavonoid pigments that give every plant its color, have been found to exhibit diversified physiologic and pharmacologic effects.

Tens of thousands of these chemical compounds have been discovered, and one of the best ways to be assured of carotenoids, beta-carotenes, lycopene, and resveratrol is to simply blend and drink, seeds, skin (with a few exceptions) and all!

Fruits and vegetables have the ability to color you healthy! Thus, to get a healthy variety of phytochemicals every day, think color. Pigments are compounds that give fruits and vegetables their color. Different pigments have different functions and react in various ways. Blending fruits and vegetables of different colors everyday gives your body a wide range of valuable nutrients (phytonutrients) that science now knows will protect you from almost every chronic disease known.

> *Red Fruits and Vegetables* are colored by a red pigment called lycopene, an antioxidant that neutralizes free radicals in the body. Lycopene has been known to assist with memory and reduce the risk of cancer. Another powerful agent found in red foods is called anthocyanin, which also serves as an antioxidant and is known to reduce heart disease. Nature's red fruits include strawberries, cranberries and watermelon. Red vegetables include red peppers, radishes and beets.

> *Orange and Yellow Fruits and Vegetables* are colored by an orange pigment called beta carotene. Carotenes contribute to photosynthesis by transmitting the light energy they absorb from chlorophyll, which gives these sunny fruits and vegetables their brilliant color. Orange and yellow fruits and vegetables are abundant in antioxidants, vitamins and phytonutrients, which are good for your skin, eyes and heart and may also decrease your risk of cancer. Experts say that beta-carotene can also delay cognitive aging and protect skin from sun damage. Nature's orange and yellow fruits include oranges, mangoes and peaches. Orange and yellow vegetables include sweet potatoes, corn and pumpkin.

> *Blue and Purple Fruits and Vegetables* are colored by a purple pigment called anthocyanin, a type of phytonutrient or plant compound, hailed for

its potential disease-fighting benefits. Studies suggest anthocyanins might help reduce the risk of heart disease, diabetes and certain types of cancer. Some evidence indicates that these purple pigments might protect our brains as we age. Blue and purple fruits include blueberries, plums and grapes. Blue and purple vegetables include eggplant, cabbage and endive.

White Fruits and Vegetables are colored by a white pigment called flavones, which contain varying amounts of phytochemicals of interest to scientists. These include allicin, an anti-fungal compound found in the garlic and onion family, and beta-glucans and lignans, which have powerful immune boosting properties. These powerful phytochemicals are also known to balance hormones, activate natural killer B and T cells, reduce the risk of colon, breast, prostate and hormone-related cancers. Nature's white fruits include bananas, pears and dates. White vegetables include onions, potatoes and cauliflower.

Eat Fermented Foods

Cultured and fermented foods have been around for thousands of years; kimchi and sauerkraut are just two examples. Most of us, unfortunately, are unaware of this lost knowledge and wonder why, even when eating an organic, raw food diet, we could still be suffering from a low to high-grade Candida infection. Candida is often caused by an imbalance of friendly bacteria in the intestinal tract, resulting in an overgrowth of fungus that ranges from mild to severe. It can also be caused by blood sugar disorders.

As we previously stated, Candida is a microbe that lives in the bloodstream and is designed to be there in a regulated fashion moderated by our blood sugar. Candida consumes blood sugar and when our blood sugar is present in normal amounts, the amount of Candida remains stable. The problem arises when the food supply becomes excessive and Candida multiplies to keep up with the excessive food demand. If a person's insulin is unable to escort the sugar out of the bloodstream, the sugar can't get out and Candida keeps blooming. What keeps the insulin from escorting sugar out is the over consumption of fat—the more fat in your diet the less effective insulin is at getting sugar out of the blood stream.

Research has shown that uptake, transport and delivery of sugar is compromised as fat intake rises. Thus, our total caloric daily intake of fat should never exceed 15% while better results can be achieved at 10%.

The long-term danger of Candida overgrowth is a compromised immune system which makes us vulnerable to almost every disease known—a underlying ecological debilitation in which most never uncover the underlying cause.

Along with following a diet low in fat and high in simple carbohydrates like fruits, leafy green vegetables and sprouts, I also recommend consuming cultured foods in the form of nuts and seeds. Cultured nuts and seeds are the best way to get your daily requirement of protein as they are pre-digested.

While the following recipe can be used for all nuts and seeds, my two favorites are sunflower seeds and almonds. I usually double the recipe because I like to eat one cup per day to assure that I'm getting adequate amounts of protein as well as probiotics. After culturing, feel free to add your favorite organic culinary herb or spice such as dillweed or curry to this recipe created by health crusader, Lou Corona…thanks Lou!

Eat Locally Grown, Seasonal Foods

Another key to a healthy diet is to eat locally and seasonally. Food grown close to home is satiated with nutrition because it is picked close to its ripened peak and is less likely to have been treated with toxic herbicides or pesticides shipped in from countries without regulations.

Eating locally and seasonally can be healthy for the environment as well. Buying foods purchased from your "food shed," loosely defined as farms within 100 miles of your home, helps to curtail global warming. Shipping and trucking food from all corners of the world uses millions of gallons of gasoline for transportation, not to mention all of the carbon dioxide it releases into the environment, just to get to the supermarket.

Produce purchased from the supermarket has been in transit or cold-stored for days or weeks, whereas produce purchased from a local farmer's market has often been picked within 24 hours of your purchase. This freshness not only affects the flavor of your food, but the nutritional value as well, which declines with time and changes in temperature.

Spending your money at a local farmer's market is important for a multitude of reasons. It not only supports your health and the environment, but it also supports the farmers in your community as well as local economy.

Many farms offer produce subscriptions, where buyers receive a weekly or monthly basket of produce, flowers, fruits, eggs, milk, meats, or any sort of different farm products. Community Supported Agriculture (CSA) is a way for the food-buying public to create a relationship with a farm and to receive a weekly basket of produce. By making a financial commitment to a farm, people become members of the CSA.

A CSA season typically runs from late spring through early fall, and correlates to Chinese medicine, where the body is seen as a microcosm of the natural world, waxing and waning with the movements of the seasons. The Chinese dietary tradition focuses on eating foods that harmonize with the changing seasons.

Autumn, for example, is a good time for loading up on warmer, heavier oily foods in preparation for the winter and cutting out most fruits. Beneficial warming foods include whole grains, cooked squashes and other root vegetables, nuts and seeds. Winter is a good time to focus on storing up energy, rest and meditation. Strengthening, warming foods like soups and stews are eaten. In the spring, the cycle begins anew. Warming, more oily and building foods are replaced by cleansing and revitalizing foods like leafy greens and sprouts to help harmonize the body with this season of rejuvenation and growth. Then, as summer begins, the diet is extremely low in fat and would consist of melons and citrus fruits, leafy greens and cool liquids.

When making choices for each changing season, I often refer to the following list.

SEASONAL FRUITS & VEGETABLES

Spring (March-May)

Avocados, bananas, cherries, artichokes, asparagus, shallots, grapefruit, lemons, mangoes, broccoli, cabbage, cauliflower, navel oranges, papayas, pineapple, celery, cucumbers, garlic, apples, plums, strawberries, leeks, lettuce, mushrooms, raspberries, watercress, potatoes, rhubarb, snap beans, spinach, squash, onions, dandelion greens, parsnips, peas, herbs, carrots, beetroots, radishes, kale, watercress, parsley.

Summer (June-August)

Apricots, blueberries, artichokes, cabbage, carrots, peas, boysenberries, cantaloupes, zucchini, cauliflower, cherries, grapefruit, grapes, honeydew, celery, corn, cucumber, lemons, nectarines, eggplant, garlic, peppers, peaches, Persian melons, strawberries, lettuce, mushrooms, okra, Valencia oranges, watermelon, onions, potatoes, spinach, gooseberries, mangoes, squash, tomatoes, watercress, radish, raspberries.

Fall (September-November)

Apples, cantaloupe, dates, artichokes, broccoli, lettuce, cranberries, grapefruit, grapes, cabbage, carrots, celery, honeydew, lemons, plums, chili peppers, cucumbers, papayas, pears, blackberries, French beans, endive, leeks, Persian melons, persimmons, figs, escarole, peppers, peas, kale, kiwi, peaches, raspberries, parsnips, onions, yams, pumpkin, lettuce, potatoes, sweet potatoes, turnips, spinach, cauliflower, sweet corn, tomatoes, squash, watercress, chestnuts, beetroot, celeriac.

Winter (December-February)

Grapefruit, lemons, kiwi, navel oranges, artichokes, broccoli, cabbage, persimmons, tangelos, Brussels sprouts, cauliflower, tangerines, pears, celery, spinach, squash, turnips, lettuce, mushrooms, potatoes, tomatoes, parsnips, rutabaga.

The following is a summary of the overarching principles you can follow to ensure optimal nourishment during every changing season:

- Spring is the season of the liver. So lower your wintery fat intake and focus on tender leafy greens and sprouts that represent the fresh new growth of this season. The greening that occurs in springtime should be represented by greens on your plate, including Swiss chard, spinach, Romaine lettuce, fresh parsley and basil.

- Summer is the season of the heart. So keep your fat intake low and focus more on a cooling fruit and vegetable diet. These foods include fruits like watermelon, strawberries, apples, pears and plums; vegetables like cucumber, tomatoes, summer squash, broccoli, cauliflower and corn; and spices and seasonings like peppermint and cilantro.

- Autumn is the season of the lung. So begin to turn towards more warming autumn harvest foods, including carrot, sweet potato, onion and garlic. Also emphasize the more warming spices and seasonings including ginger, peppercorns and mustard seeds. Begin to increase your fat intake.

- Winter is the season of the kidney. Turn even more exclusively toward warming foods as raw foods tend to cool the body. Focus more on foods that take the longest to grow, such as root vegetables, carrot, potato, beans, onions, ginger and garlic. Increase your fat intake to 15-20%.

Follow the Circadian Rhythm

Your body follows certain daily cycles known as the circadian rhythm. Circadian refers to the regular recurrence of cycles of activity that occur approximately every 24 hours, or one full day. The rhythm is linked to the light-dark cycle. While sleep cycles are the most common studied by science, it has also been found that if a person's daily eating patterns are in tune with these naturally occurring rhythms, they will notice a tremendous increase in their overall health, energy and wellbeing.

There are three cycles associated with the circadian rhythm: (1) consumption (eating and digesting), (2) assimilation (extracting nutrients and assimilating) and (3) elimination (purging and releasing). Each has its own eight-hour period during which its activities are the most heightened.

The *consumption* cycle is from 12 noon until 8pm. This is the time when the body is most capable of efficiently taking in and digesting food.

The *assimilation* cycle is from 8pm to 4am. This is the time the body is extracting nutrients and assimilating what it needs.

The *elimination* cycle is from 4am to 12 noon. This is the time when the body is gathering wastes and preparing them for removal.

Step 1: The Consumption Cycle

Food should be eaten between 12 noon until 8pm. This is when your body is in the consumption cycle. The consumption cycle occurs when the body is predisposed to digesting food and allotting the energy to do so. In fact, Chinese medicine has long taught that our digestive fire increases and decreases according to the position of the sun. Thus, because the sun is at its greatest intensity from noon until 3pm, these three hours are the most optimal time to consume the majority of our food.

Step 2: The Assimilation Cycle

Food should *not* be eaten between 8pm and 4am. This is when your body switches from the consumption cycle over to the assimilation cycle and starts the process of extracting and assimilating the nutrients from the food you've eaten during the day. Hence, after the food you've consumed has been digested, energy is needed to extract and utilize the nutrients the body requires for optimal function. If food is eaten after 8pm, your body is forced out of the assimilation cycle and back to the consumption cycle, diverting energy away from proper nutrient extraction and uptake and stressing your digestive system.

Step 3: The Elimination Cycle

Food other than fruit should *not* be eaten between 4am to 12 noon. This is when your body is in the elimination cycle. Food consumed prior to the completion of the elimination cycle not only severely retards the process of eliminating the accumulated wastes from the body; it also throws the rhythm of the three cycles into turmoil. The best way to flush out the accumulated waste during this cycle is to drink lots of ionized alkaline water (about one quart) upon waking. Then just eat fruit until noon. Consuming fruit during this time does not disrupt the elimination cycle because the sugar component in fruit is a carbohydrate in its simplest form, glucose. Thus it requires absolutely zero digestive energy to break down the sugar molecule and make use of the energy. Fruit also holds the plant kingdom's honor of being nature's greatest food for cleansing waste from the physical body.

Food Combining

Food combining is the term that emphasizes the importance of properly combining the types of foods you eat, as well as that of properly timing their consumption. While certain food combining principles are as ancient as the Mosaic Covenant (the Jewish law requiring the separating of meat and milk), some of today's top nutritional researchers report that some foods are digested differently, thus should be eaten separately and at different times.

They report that the most important rule of food combining is not to mix a meal of carbohydrate-rich foods such as bread, rice, cereals and carrots with protein-rich foods such as meat, milk, eggs, beans, nuts and seeds. Another important rule is to always eat fruit alone and wait 20-30 minutes before eating another meal so that the fruit has time to pass through the stomach, since fruit does not require digestion in the stomach with the help of gastric juices.

According to the studies of Dr. Herbert M. Shelton, the father of food combining, there are sound physiological reasons for not eating foods that are incompatible combinations:

- Starchy foods require an alkaline digestive medium, which is supplied initially in the mouth by the enzyme ptyalin.

- Protein foods require an acid medium for digestion, which is supplied by hydrochloric acid.

In short, acids and alkalis neutralize each other. Therefore, if you eat a starch with a protein, digestion is impaired or completely arrested, and undigested food can cause various kinds of digestive disorders. It becomes soil for unfriendly bacteria, which ferment and decompose, making poisonous by-products. One of these by-products is alcohol, which destroys or inhibits nerve function. Undigested food plays havoc with the nerves of the digestive tract, suspending their vital action such that constipation may well be the end result.

While there is currently a shortage of medical research supporting these theories, there are thousands of testimonials by people who claim that they have experienced significant improvements from carefully combining foods. Some of these are: weight loss, improved digestive related health conditions including acid reflux, bloating, stomach ache, gas emissions and fatigue experienced after eating.

If there were only three food combining rules to follow, mine would be: (1) don't mix meat with dairy (i.e., a hamburger with cheese), (2) don't mix carbohydrates and proteins, (meat and potatoes) and (3) eat fruit alone, with the exception of green leafy greens. It's as simple as that!

Mindful Under-eating & Periodic Fasting

The main function of blood cells is to distribute oxygen to every part of the body. But when we overeat, our cells are forced to act mainly as the body's waste removal system. Thus, instead of supplying the body with needed oxygen, blood cells must first get rid of unprocessed food waste; waste that ends up getting stored in various parts of the body. Then, as we continue to overeat and our bodies never have the opportunity to properly eliminate these stored toxins, our energy decreases and disease sets in.

Recent studies (conducted at the Laboratory of Neurosciences, National Institute on Aging Gerontology Research Center, Laboratory of Neurosciences and Comparative Medicine, National Institute on Aging, Department of Human Genetics and Department of Neuroscience, John Hopkins University School of Medicine) have shown that both under-eating due to calorie restrictions and intermittent fasting, with maintained vitamin and mineral intake, can extend lifespan and increase resistance to disease.

It was also discovered that mindful under-eating has a positive effect on brain function and debilitating diseases such as Alzheimer's, Parkinson's and strokes due to the fact that it can protect neurons (a cell that transmits nerve impulses) against degeneration. In addition, under-eating can stimulate the production of new neurons from stem cells, which may increase the ability of the brain to resist aging and restore function after an injury.

Research shows that healthful effects of intermittent fasting and under-eating could be the result of a cellular stress response that stimulates the production of proteins that enhance resistance to metabolic and oxidative insults. It is assumed that this sort of stress may also have similar favorable effects on brain and muscle tissue by stimulating regeneration of brain and muscle cells via activation of stress proteins and the production of growth factors.

While vitamins, minerals and antioxidants may improve the health of the brain, it was shown that the major factor for brain health is an increase in the time between meals. Studying a range of organisms, from yeast and roundworms to rodents and monkeys, showed that their maximum lifespan could be increased by up to 50%, simply by under-feeding them or reducing their calorie intake. They also discovered that under-eating reduced the incidence of age-related cancer, cardiovascular disease and immune deficiencies in rodents while a high calorie intake or over-feeding increased the risk for all degenerative diseases, such as cardiovascular disease, various types of cancers, type-II diabetes and stroke.

It was suggested that if we would eat only one meal per day and periodically fast, we could diminish degenerative disease, greatly reducing the incidence of stroke, as well as Alzheimer's and Parkinson's disease—three devastating syndromes that currently plague our society.

WATER—The Alkaline Drink

Water is the gift of life. Every life form that exists on earth was conceived in and raised out of water. Our bodies took form in a water sac held within our mother's womb; once the nine-month gestation period was complete, the water broke and we were born; born of water. As stated earlier, our body, like our planetary body, is mostly water. Every cell, like the fish in the sea, swims and bathes itself in water. Water is everywhere and flows throughout everything. We bathe in it, play in it, swim in it, get baptized in it, cook in it, and drink it. Therefore, it's logical to conclude that every aspect of maintaining a healthy body exists within the structure of a water molecule.

A Water Molecule

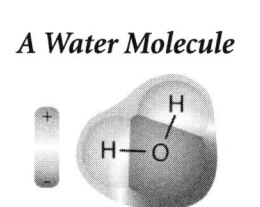

A water molecule is like the Holy Trinity held within the chemistry of our physical existence. It's a compound of hydrogen and oxygen: 2 parts hydrogen and 1 part oxygen. Hydrogen, which makes up 75% of the universe by volume, has the highest energy content per unit weight of any known fuel. Yet it never occurs by itself in nature—it always combines with other elements such as oxygen (for water) and carbon (for fossil fuel). Unfortunately, the waters of our body, like the waters of our earth, have become hydrogen-depleted, predisposing us to a life of suffering from various diseases that originate from an ecological breakdown.

The good news is that clinical tests conducted in Japan proved that regular drinking of hydrogen-rich water may result in *curing, improving and preventing* many diseases while slowing down the aging process. The key to life is proper hydration.

F. Batmanghelidj, M.D., author of *Your Body's Many Cries For Water,* proved in his years of research that Unintentional Chronic Dehydration (UCD) contributes to and even produces pain and many degenerative diseases that can be prevented and treated by increasing water intake on a regular basis. With the right *quality* and *quantity* of water, he believes that you can even cure the sick. He says, "You're not sick; you're thirsty. Don't treat thirst with medication."

Drink Ionized Alkaline Water

When life began on earth, streams of water flowed over rocky surfaces, causing an interaction of life forces now known as ionization. Ionization is the process of converting a molecule into an ion by adding or removing negatively charged particles such as electrons. This highly charged ionized water is characterized by groups of small cluster-size molecules that are hydrogen-rich, having the ability to penetrate the cell membrane, enabling nutrients to easily enter and wastes to effortlessly exit. While the source of the water we drink is important, the structure of that water, being hydrogen-poor or hydrogen-rich is the most significant key.

Water becomes de-ionized and hydrogen-depleted as a result of pollution. In fact, the waters of our earth have become so polluted that they are now considered harmful. It has been suggested that water pollution is the leading worldwide cause of death, and that it accounts for the deaths of more than 14,000 people daily. The Centers for Disease Control and Prevention (CDC) reports that 900,000 to 1,000,000 Americans will get sick from drinking contaminated water this year alone. They, amongst major medical journals, say that good ole' fashioned tap water can be downright lethal. It has been shown to trigger a massive heart attack, riddle your body with cancer, make your bones crumble, infect your body with deadly parasites and much more. The CDC reports, "what comes out of your faucet is not water...it's a toxic soup of chemicals, bacteria, viruses and heavy metals!"

Fortunately, a water processing technology from Japan that was developed in 1965 creates water the way nature originally designed it to be. This ionization process reduces the size of a normal water molecule cluster by at least two-thirds. Where tap water is typically 12-15 molecules per cluster, as a result of the electrolysis process, this water has smaller clusters of 5-6 water molecules, making it hydrogen-rich and super-hydrating; water that promotes healing. These small clusters of water are called Hexagonal Water.

The significance of creating smaller water molecule clusters is that, as we previously stated, it makes it easier for them to penetrate the cell membrane, which enhances tissue repair, nutrient absorption and waste removal. Smaller water clusters recreate nature's most perfect water. It is naturally oxygenated, thus it automatically increases the body's oxygen levels. Its super-hydrating micro-cluster molecules, fortified by millions of age-defying, mineralized, antioxidants, neutralize free radicals and boost your metabolism. They also remove acid wastes from the "waters" of your body while alkalizing every part of your internal terrain. It also accelerates the release of harmful chemicals, heavy metals, toxins...and even fat cells.

Dr. Mu Shik John, researcher and author of *The Water Puzzle and the Hexagonal Key* states: "Hexagonal water, comprised of small molecular units or ring-shaped clusters, moves easily within the cellular matrix of the body, helping with nutrient absorption and waste removal. It aids metabolic processes, supports the immune system, contributes to lasting vitality and acts as a carrier of dissolved oxygen. It can provide alkaline minerals to the body and it helps in the more efficient removal of acidic wastes. Drinking hexagonal water takes us in the direction of health. It supports long life and freedom from disease. Biological organisms prefer hexagonal water."

Following decades of research, this Japanese technology is being used extensively in hospitals, industries and homes all around the world. Regular tap water is first purified, and then given an electrical charge that ionizes it, which causes positive and negative ions to split into two distinct acid and alkaline streams. The acid water aids in treating skin disorders and the alkaline water aids in neutralizing excess acids while alkalizing the internal environment of your body.

The Japanese Association of Preventive Medicine for Adult Diseases (the equivalent to the U.S. FDA) has even approved this unique patented water processor as a medical device for its effectiveness in assisting the body to rebuild itself from dehydration and many illnesses and diseases linked to the effects of dehydration. Some of the areas that people have noticed improvements in their health include arthritis, chronic fatigue, leg cramps, migraines, and diabetes. Also heartburn, poor circulation, gout, tendonitis, high blood pressure, high cholesterol, asthma, skin rashes, dermatitis, psoriasis, weight issues, diarrhea, indigestion, heart disease, allergies, constipation, stomach ulcers, hepatitis, cancer, and many more areas have had considerable positive results.

As I see it, dehydration is but a reflection of the droughts of the earth, which occurs when a region (organs and glands) notes a deficiency in its water supply. Thus, when you drink ionized alkaline water *the rainforest way,* you will no long suffer from famines and related diseases that come from malnutrition and shortages in electricity production. Here's what I mean.

Rainforests are forests characterized by high levels of rainfall, raining over 80 inches each year. Tropical rainforests have been called the "jewels of the Earth" as they are havens for millions of green plants that generate much of the Earth's oxygen. In a rainforest, plants and

Your inner rainforest will flourish when you drink ionized alkaline water the rainforest way!

microorganisms flourish because the rains come down in a constant mist instead of sporadic downpours. Thus, when you drink 4-6 ounces of water every 30 minutes every day *the rainforest way* and consume lots of greens, your inner rainforest will also flourish.

Take A Detox Bath

When you get sick with a cold or other illness, your body's natural defense is to produce a fever. With an elevated body temperature, your immune system is able to work at a heightened level so that your body is able to fight against any viruses or bacteria more effectively. Elevated body temperatures also increase the speed and efficiency of blood circulation, thereby increasing the supply of blood to the "battle zones" in the body while speeding the removal of acid waste. The higher body temperature also facilitates recovery from fatigue or stress. This is why wounded wild animals have been seen bathing in hot springs in the mountains, using their instinctual wisdom to speed up healing by soaking themselves in hot mineral water.

In order to take full therapeutic advantage of a hot bath, you must stay in the bath for 20 minutes or longer. While hot baths help to accelerate the *Get Clean* process, when you take a Celtic Sea Salt® bath, the benefits are astounding. Not only will an enormous amount of toxins be released through the skin during the bath, but the highly charged minerals from the salt will also be absorbed, helping to alkalinize your internal terrain. Just be sure the water you're bathing in has been filtered.

It has been noted that a person can get rid of heavy metals such as lead, mercury, arsenic, amalgam and calcium because the whole crystal salt facilitates the breakup of their molecular structures. Salt water therapy can also assist in releasing any calcium build up, but for the body to get rid of these deposits, it has to first metabolize them. Even animal proteins, which are difficult to break down and eliminate, will be eliminated through the urine due to the strong structural formation of the crystal salt.

Most bath salts you'll find on store shelves, however, do not hold the cleansing and regenerating power of Celtic Bath Salts. Their crystals are truly "diamonds in the rough." Thus, for the ultimate bath, pour about two pounds of Celtic Salt Crystals into a clean, standard-sized tub. If your bathtub is not standard size, you can calculate the amount of salt required by using the formula of 1.28-ounces of salt per gallon of water. This generates a 1% solution.

Add just enough hot water to cover the crystals and wait for about 10 minutes, or until they have almost dissolved. Now fill the bathtub, but resist the temptation to run a steaming-hot bath. Water closer to your normal body temperature will create less stress on your body. Simply fill the bathtub, keeping the water comfortably warm, but not too hot. Remain in the bath for 20-30 minutes. You may want to keep adding hot water to maintain the steady water temperature. Be sure to drink lots of ionized alkaline water while you are bathing. If you begin to feel faint or weak, don't stay any longer; shower the salts off and towel dry.

Because the hot salt bath makes demands on the circulatory system, the process of detoxification may make you feel a little weak for a short time afterwards (10-15 minutes). Note that if you have a heart condition, poor circulation or high blood pressure, you might consider a footbath instead of a full bath.

Hot & Cold Water Therapy

Ancient civilizations have long recognized the healing power of using alternating hot and cold water. As far back as the 4th Century, the great Greek physician Hippocrates prescribed this type of therapy for its beneficial healing effects. The Romans even built communal baths because they believed in the healing power of hot and cold applications. These alternating applications have been found to be helpful for almost every conceivable healing process known.

Hot and cold water assists better circulation of blood in the body, which helps to decrease inflammation, get more white blood cells circulating and stimulates the white blood cells to become more effective against infection. Chronic conditions such as high blood pressure, kidney disease, diabetes and chronic infections benefit from hot and cold hydrotherapy, which stimulates the body's immune system and improves the vital energy in the body. Acute conditions such as headaches or menstrual cramps benefit from alternating hot and cold applications to relieve pain and discomfort.

Alternating hot and cold baths are good for treating hands and feet. With water as hot as you can stand it in one bowl, ice water in the other, put hands or feet in the hot water for one minute, then plunge into the cold for 20 seconds. Then back into hot and cold again until a total of 10 minutes have been spent doing this, ending with the plunge into the ice water. This process has been reported to be beneficial for arthritic joints and tired, aching feet, plus the alternating hot and cold stimulates circulation.

An alternating hot and cold footbath is also great in promoting circulation in the legs, helping with varicose veins, insomnia, headaches, high blood pressure as well as generating an overall sense of wellbeing. The best thing is, it is easily accomplished in the comfort of your own home.

Colonic Hydrotherapy

When you begin eating a diet high in plant foods, flushing out the accumulated toxic waste from your colon is of utmost importance.

Recently, the subject of alimentary toxemia was discussed in London before the Royal Society of Medicine by 57 leading physicians of Great Britain. Among the speakers were eminent surgeons, physicians and specialists in various branches of medicine. According to the Royal Society of Medicine, 90% of all chronic diseases are due to an infection of the gastrointestinal tract. It should be understood that these findings are not mere theories, but are the results of demonstrations in actual practice by some of the most eminent physicians of our time.

While they do not claim that alimentary toxemia is the only cause of disease, they do, however, recognize that when the colon is clean and normal, we are basically disease-free. But left to stagnate, it will distill the poisons of decay, fermentation and putrefaction into the blood, poisoning virtually every tissue, gland and organ system. These poisons infiltrate brain cells, along with our nervous system, contributing to depression and irritability. They also poison the heart so that we are weak and listless, poison the lungs so that the breath is foul, poison the digestive organs so that we are distressed and bloated, and poison the blood so that the skin is sallow and unhealthy. In essence, their findings were that most of our diseases are rooted in alimentary toxemia.

From this extensive study, Dr. W. Bezley reported, *"There are a few phases of cardiovascular trouble (disease of heart and blood vessels) with which disorder of some part of the alimentary tract is not causatively associated."* Dr. Lane reported that rheumatoid arthritis is the direct result of intestinal toxicity. He stated, *"I do not believe it is possible for either of these diseases to obtain a foothold except in the presence of stasis."* Dr. Lane went so far as to say, *"Auto-intoxication plays so large a part in the development of disease of the female genito-urinary apparatus, that they may be regarded by the gynecologist as a product of intestinal stasis."*

It is now estimated that 80% of our immune system is located in or around the digestive system, especially the large intestine, thus keeping our colon clean is of utmost importance. This means that until the colon is thoroughly cleansed and the toxins removed, nutrients will not absorb properly and digestion will be hindered. This leads to constipation and alimentary toxemia, creating uncomfortable maladies such as gas, bloating, IBS, headaches, bad breath, allergy symptoms, PMS, fatigue, depression, irritability, frequent infections, and weight gain.

In essence, the colon is the sewage system of our house (body), but by neglect and abuse it can become a backed-up toxic cesspool. Therefore, cleansing the colon through various herbal cleansing formulas along with colon hydrotherapy is vitally important. And, through the years, colon hydrotherapy has become one of the most popular ways to clean out the alimentary poisons from the colon.

Colon hydrotherapy, also known as a colonic, flushes the colon with gallons of warm filtered water by a professional colon hydrotherapist or, they can simply be self-administered in the privacy of your home by using a home colonic board.

The cost of a professional colonic treatment is about $60 per session. The patient changes into a gown and lies on a padded table so that the colon hydrotherapist can insert a sterile, double lumen tube gently into the anus. The colon is then gently flushed with repeated doses of warmed filtered water, which loosens waste stuck in the colon and filters it out through a tube system.

The cost of a home colonic board is around $300. Dr. Bernard Jensen, one of the world's leading authorities on colon health, recommends at least two to three colonic irrigations per week during his seven-day cleansing program. He recommends this seven-day series five times per year for the first year. Once the colon is cleansed after the first year, he then recommends the seven-day session once per year for maintenance. Setting up a self-administering colonic irrigation at home will save you hundreds of dollars. After your fifth session, you will have paid for your board while using the board for many years thereafter. A very wise investment indeed.

Following *The Four "Fuel" Groups* is simple and easy. Better yet, it's a great way to build that strong foundation toward becoming the healthy, happier you that you were designed to be. Just know that when you start aligning yourself with the four elemental forces of nature—air, fire, earth, and water—the process is steady but sure. And all you have to do to begin the journey to that healthier, happier, more balanced *ecological you* is to start by taking one alkalizing bite at a time!

CHAPTER EIGHT

The Get Clean Go Green
EcoDiet Program

Now that you have a basic understanding of your body as a living ecosystem and how ecosystems thrive and how they die, let's take a look at the program that I believe will assist you on becoming that healthier more alkaline *you* that you were designed to be. To summarize the program, let's consider the seven most important alkalizing secrets to incorporate in your *Get Clean Go Green EcoDiet*.

THE SECRETS OF AN ALKALINE ENVIRONMENT

Secret #1—Just Breathe Nothing else will alkalize you quicker than breathing. The sheer movement of breathing out carbon dioxide eliminates acids and alkalizes the blood. To return to a perfect state of health or simply burn up any extra body fat that you may be wearing, consider a series of deep breathing exercises. Use any breath technique that fits your particular lifestyle each day. Bounce on a rebounder (mini-trampoline), take a fast walk, bend, stretch, walk, do yoga, qigong, jog…just breathe and do lots of it!

Secret #2—Eat Light Medical studies have shown that exposure to sunlight every day without sun block increases our vitamin D intake as well as decreases the risk of colorectal cancer by more than 65% and breast cancer by 50%. It has also been shown that sunlight increases the number of white blood cells, which plays the leading role in defending against invasions by bacteria and foreign organisms. Sunlight is your friend. Just be sure to use wisdom when it comes to exposing yourself to the sun.

Secret #3—Drink Ionized Alkaline Water Medical studies show that ionized alkaline water has powerful antioxidant properties, better than vitamins A, C, E, beta carotene and selenium, which substantially improves your body's defense against disease. An alkaline water ionizer is more than a water filter; it is a special type of water system that changes the structure of water to an ionized alkaline state. It is this ionized alkaline state that is reported to create so many healthy benefits. So drink lots of it every day, and the best kept alkalizing water secret is to drink 3-4 ounces every half hour, *the rainforest way.*

Secret #4—Get Clean Cleansing your entire intestinal tract of undigested accumulated acid waste, mucoid plaque and other toxins, is of primary importance to your alkalizing *Get Clean Go Green EcoDiet* process. It has been proven that, over time, as acid waste from undigested food particles builds up in the intestinal tract, in order to protect itself from the acids, the body produces a mucoid plaque lining on the intestinal wall. This plaque inhibits the intake of nutrients and the proper elimination of wastes, which fosters the overgrowth of unfriendly bacteria. So *Get Clean*, then restore your intestines with lots of friendly bacteria. You'll be glad you did!

Secret #5—Go Green Eat plenty of raw, phytonutrient-rich, organic green leafy salads and/or drink lots of freshly prepared green juices every day. Along with your salads and green juices, you'll also want to consume organic celery and green powders, such as barley green or a combination of greens. Celery is loaded with organic sodium, which neutralizes acids, making it one of the most alkalizing foods you can consume, and organic green powders are some of the most nutrient dense foods on the planet.

Secret #6—Eat Lots of Fruit in Season A diet high in raw, enzyme-rich, organic fruit, which is easily converted into glucose, is necessary in order to attain high levels of oxygen. If your blood is low in glucose, you'll tend to be a shallow breather because the extra oxygen simply cannot be used. So follow the circadian rhythm and begin every day with a fruit breakfast and/or a fruit superfood smoothie. Try a grapefruit or two first thing in the morning as they are very alkalizing. But if it's wintertime and cold where you live and fruits are out of season, shift to a more warming seasonal diet.

Secret #7—Chew the Fat The best way to make sure you're getting enough fatty acids every day is to eat foods such as an avocado or a handful of sprouted nuts and seeds. In other words, if you *chew the fat,* you'll tend to keep your daily fat consumption around 10% of your total caloric intake, which has been found to be the healthiest amount required. If you use oil on a salad or otherwise, use it sparingly and make sure it's organic and cold pressed. Just remember these two rules: (1) the more fruit you eat, the less fat you should consume and (2) the less fruit you eat, the more fat you can consume.

Now that you have an understanding of the importance of maintaining a proper acid/alkaline balance and have stopped burning the wrong types of food for fuel into your internal environment, it's time to *Get Clean* and *Go Green*. There are essentially two parts to the *Get Clean Go Green EcoDiet* program. The first part is to *Get Clean;* that is, to clean all of the accumulated toxic chemicals and acid waste out of your entire system. The second part is to *Go Green;* that is, to burn the right types of food for fuel into your internal environment. So first, let's *Get Clean.*

PART ONE

THE "GET CLEAN" PROGRAM

Like changing the oil in your car, cleansing your body all of the accumulated toxic chemicals, heavy metals and acid waste has the potential to eliminate what I call an "ecological breakdown" and what others call disease. Some have even found that when the accumulated toxic wastes are removed and you fuel the body with a diet high in alkaline foods, the body naturally heals itself.

Medical science now acknowledges this fact. Reports show that up to 85% or more of all adult Americans suffer from some sort of intestinal disorder. Intestinal disorders are created when the digestive and eliminative systems are sluggish and not working properly to rid the body of putrefied waste that builds up in the small intestines and colon. The resulting toxins are then absorbed into the bloodstream and are carried back into every part of the body, especially the liver and spleen. This process of self-poisoning is called *autointoxication.*

Because of a sluggish intestinal tract, the body ends up poisoning itself with its own wastes and toxins instead of carrying out its designed purpose of eliminating them. As this putrefied waste continues to build up in the intestines, the intestinal ecology becomes a breeding ground that encourages the rapid growth of huge colonies of toxin-producing, disease-promoting bacteria, which can result in one or more forms of serious illnesses or chronic degenerative diseases.

"And we have made of ourselves living cesspools, and driven doctors to invent names for our diseases."

– Plato

"Poor health is caused by toxic (acid) overload because everything is out of whack and cannot function properly."

–The Journal of Longevity

"The countless names of illnesses do not really matter. What does matter is that they all come from the same root cause... too much tissue acid waste in the body."

– Theodore A. Baroody, N.D., D.C., Ph.D.,
author of *Alkalize or Die*

"Every disease, no matter what name it is known by Medical Science, is Constipation! A clogging up of the entire pipe system of the human body. Any special symptom is therefore merely an extraordinary local constipation by more accumulated mucus at this particular place. Special accumulation points are the tongue, the stomach and particularly the entire digestive tract. This last is the real and deeper cause of bowel constipation. The average person has as much as ten pounds of un-eliminated feces in the bowels continually, poisoning the blood stream and the entire system. Think of it!"

– Professor Arnold Ehret,
author of *Rational Fasting*

So what does it mean to Get Clean?

- *Get Clean* means to cleanse all of the toxic chemicals and accumulated acid wastes from the waters of your body.

How about Getting Lean?

- Research at Stanford University in Palo Alto, California reports, *"Just as acid build-up in the body causes rapid weight gain, de-acidifying those fat cells causes the weight to virtually fall off."*

After years of alternative health research, I am now convinced that the first step towards regaining the proper acid-alkaline balance is the complete and thorough cleansing of the intestinal tract. Because most of us have spent years feeding our bodies with the wrong types of food for fuel, I am now also convinced that a 14-day intestinal cleanse should be a must for everyone two to three times a year.

At first, I was concerned about fasting or cleansing too much. But then, after discovering that certain tiny water animals alternately fed one week and starved the next during their entire life, lived five times longer than those that were fed all the time, I had no more concern. This is when I discovered that the key to health, is to *cleanse* and *feed;* that is, to *Get Clean* and *Go Green!*

> *"Fasting and natural diet, though essentially unknown (in today's U.S.) as a therapy, should be the first treatment when someone discovers that she or he has a medical problem. It should not be applied only to the most advanced cases, as is present practice. Whether the patient has a cardiac condition, hypertension, autoimmune disease, fibroids, or asthma, he or she must be informed that fasting and natural, plant-based diets are a viable alternative to conventional therapy, and an effective one. The time may come when not offering this substantially more effective nutritional approach will be considered malpractice."*

> – Joel Fuhrman, M.D., author of
> *Fasting And Eating For Health*

STEP #1: THE "GET CLEAN" PRECLEANSE

To begin, it's important to be aware that if you've never cleansed before, chances are that you might feel headachy or even experience flu-like symptoms. These types of symptoms indicate that your body is dumping stored-up toxins and acids and your bloodstream is overloaded with acid waste. Taking a hot detox clay bath or a bath consisting of 1 cup apple cider vinegar, 1 cup Celtic Bath Salts and 2 tablespoons ground ginger or any form of sweat-induced therapy will assist this process greatly.

Another way to decrease an acid overload is to follow a precleanse diet along with a precleanse supplementation program for a few weeks, a month or even two months before going into deeper levels of cleansing.

If you've been eating the Standard American Diet (SAD) for years and/or your alkaline reserves are low (according to the internal acid rain study as outlined in Chapter 4), you'll definitely want to start cleansing slowly. Simply enjoy the precleanse diet along with the precleanse supplements until your alkaline reserves are back to normal. Long term, you'll be glad you did!

Week One: Eat an all plant-based organic diet: 20% slightly acid-forming foods such as grains and beans, and 80% alkaline-forming foods such as fruits and vegetables—20% cooked and 80% raw. Eliminate all fats from your diet with the exception of an avocado or a small amount of cold pressed organic olive or grapeseed oil with lemon juice on your salad. Drink several quarts of ionized alkaline water *the rainforest way* throughout the day. Take digestive enzymes with each meal along with the precleanse supplements, as outlined in the "PreCleanse" and "EcoCleanse" Supplement Section.

Week Two: Eat an all plant-based organic raw food diet such as fresh fruits, green-leafy salads, vegetables, and juices with the exclusion of: grains, beans, nuts, or seeds. Follow the same precleanse supplement program as week one.

The Gallbladder Flush: Consider doing a gallbladder flush twice a day during week two; first thing in the morning and last thing at night. Drinking 2-3 quarts of freshly-prepared organic apple juice during the day also helps soften any gallstones you may have, which will greatly assist in eliminating them.

The Gallbladder Flush Recipe: In a blender, add 1/3-cup organic extra virgin olive oil with 2/3 cup fresh lemon or grapefruit juice, 3 peeled garlic cloves, 1" piece fresh ginger, and a dash of cayenne pepper. For a more palatable drink top off with 1/4 cup orange juice. For best results, lie on your right side with knees to chest for 10-15 minutes immediately after drinking this mixture. The mixture will then move up the gallbladder duct and into the gallbladder and soften any gallstones you may have.

The Gallbladder/Liver Flush Juice: You can also dissolve the stagnation and stones in your gallbladder and liver over time with a specific apple/beet/ginger juice recipe listed in the following "EcoJuice" Fast section.

PRECLEANSE SUPPLEMENTS

The Alkalizer a concentrated electrolyte formula your body depends on to assist in rebuilding your alkaline reserves with the most essential alkaline minerals possible. Electrolytes also helps to remove toxic acids, maintain fluid balance in cells, balance pH levels, normalize hormone secretion, nerve conduction and various other important functions. Electrolytes have three roles: (1) they provide structural materials for bones and other connective tissue, (2) they act as catalysts or supporting the role of enzymes in physiological processes and (3) they allow electrical impulses to move along the nerves. This product also contains inulin, a group of naturally occurring polysaccharides produced by many types of plants. Inulin is known to work as a prebiotic, meaning that it is a great food source for the growth of friendly bacteria. Because inulin is not digested or absorbed in the stomach, it goes to the bowels where beneficial bacteria use it to multiply.

Probiotics a formula that restores the friendly bacteria to your intestinal tract that have most likely been destroyed from a diet high in acid-forming foods and/or pharmaceutical drugs such as steroids and antibiotics. Friendly bacteria, also known as probiotics, are living microorganisms that provide an array of health benefits. The types of bacteria present in the right amounts are essential for a strong immunity. When friendly bacteria are not present the way nature intended, our immunity lowers and our line of defense is lost against unfriendly microorganisms and parasites.

Replacing beneficial bacteria through probiotic supplementation is extremely helpful in reestablishing a healthy intestinal ecology. Because the intestinal tract is slightly alkaline, when looking for the right formula, look for a product that contains *bifidobacterium* strains normally found in a healthy intestinal tract. Many probiotic formulas on the market are primarily lactobacillus such as *lactobacillus acidophilus*, which are acid-producing and should only be used to help destroy an overgrowth of Candida or other unfriendly bacteria. Probiotics, such as bifidobacterium, are more alkaline-producing and natural to the human intestines. The right balance of probiotics has shown to have the power to eliminate waste and toxins from the intestines, improve digestion and nutrient absorption, work against harmful molds, yeast, fungi and viruses and strengthen our immunity.

> **Note** If you were to add the right amount and type of probiotics to a polluted pond or lake, they would clean up the water and remember...your body is made up of mostly water!

Herbal Intestinal Cleanse an herbal formula that will begin to soften and break up toxic waste material while detoxifying cells. An herbal combination that works well for this includes plantain, cascara sagrada, barberry, peppermint, sheep sorrel, fennel seed, ginger root, myrrh gum, red raspberry, rhubarb root, goldenseal, and lobelia. This herbal formula, along with herbal intestinal nutrition, prepares the mucoid plaque for removal and neutralizes stored intestinal toxins such as pesticides, drugs, pathogenic microorganisms and even some parasites. When this plaque is removed, the lymphatic drainage points open, which in turn allows the toxins and sludge to be dumped from all areas of the body. It also helps to cleanse the liver, skin, lungs, kidneys along with other body tissues. In addition, it allows the 22 enzymes secreted by the intestines to reach the food we eat and complete the digestive processes and assists the absorption of nutrients.

Digestive Enzymes a formula taken with every meal that contains specific enzymes to help break down fats, carbohydrates and proteins. Enzymes are one of the most essential elements in our body and most people are enzyme deficient due to an acidic diet high in processed, cooked foods. When a person's digestive system isn't functioning optimally, digestive enzymes help to break down the foods you eat, releasing nutrients for energy production and cell growth and repair. (Digestive enzymes can also be taken in-between meals to break down undigested food particles in the intestines.)

The Directions

The Alkalizer (Prebiotic)
Take 2-4 tablespoons a day in juice or water.

Probiotics
Take 6 capsules on an empty stomach with *The Alkalizer* first thing in the morning for one month then 3 capsules thereafter for 3 months.

Herbal Intestinal Cleanse
4-6 capsules 3-5 times a day on an empty stomach.

Digestive Enzymes
Take 6 capsules with every meal and 3 to 6 capsules in-between meals.

Note To purchase these and all of the recommended supplemental products that follow, please refer to the resource section in the back of this book.

Now that you've precleansed and you're on your way to becoming a healthier more alkaline *you*, to go deeper into the cleansing process, the next step is to do a 14-day intestinal cleanse while you *drink your way to wellness*.

STEP #2: DRINK YOUR WAY TO WELLNESS

Water is nature's greatest solvent. This means that water has the power to dissolve and clean the acid waste out of your body in the most efficient way possible, especially when that water is ionized alkaline water. Dr. Robert Young, microbiologist and author of *The pH Miracle for Diabetes* says, "The best way to get acid out of your body is to wash it out. The best way to wash it out is to provide plenty of water to do the job."

The reason I promote drinking ionized alkaline water is that ionized water is highly charged with negative ions and acids are charged with positive ions. This means that the negatively-charged ions will attract the positively-charged ions, i.e., heavy metals and toxic chemicals, to them and carry them out of the body. In other words, *if you can change the way you drink, you can change the way you feel*. This is because water is the basis of all life, thus the right kind of water holds the key to transforming "that which is no longer life back into life."

F. Batmaghelidj, M.D., and author of *Water: For Health, for Healing, for Life* reports, *"You're not sick; you're thirsty. Don't treat thirst with medication!"* No real miracles. Just common sense. You're dehydrated!

Dehydration, viewed from an eco-body perspective, is but an internal drought that takes place from a lack of water. These droughts can occur within a particular region (organs and glands) of the body and is one of the main causes of disease. Therefore, the solution to such an ecological breakdown is to *drink your way to wellness*. This means that when you drink lots of ionized alkaline water every day *the rainforest way*, your body (your earth) will no long suffer from droughts and famines along with their related ecological breakdowns.

Along with drinking adequate amounts of water, try drinking 1-2 quarts of freshly-prepared organic vegetable juices every day. Freshly-prepared vegetable and fruit juice is another great way to solve your acid overload and bring health back into your internal environment. Fruits and vegetables are loaded with electrolytes. Thus together, alkaline ionized water and freshly-prepared juice make a powerful healing and rejuvenating team.

So go ahead…*drink your way to wellness*…I did, and so can you! Take the 21-day *drink your way to wellness* challenge and try it for yourself. Flush those acids out of your body! Drink 4-6 ounces of ionized alkaline water and freshly-prepared vegetable and fruit juice every 30 minutes with the goal of consuming 1-ounce of water and juice for every pound of body weight for 21 days.

This means that if you weigh 120 pounds, you would consume a total of 120-ounces (approximately 1 gallon) of water and freshly-prepared vegetable juice every day. Just be sure to always drink your liquids *the rainforest way*. If you do, you may just turn your ecological breakdown around.

> **Note** When juicing, be sure to use organic or biodynamic produce when possible. If, for some reason, you're unable to find organic produce and are forced to use commercially-grown produce, just be sure to use a product called "Veggie Wash®" that will remove wax, soil and agricultural chemicals.

The 21-Day "EcoJuice" Program

The "EcoCleanse" Drink and "EcoCleanse" Herbs are to be taken during the 14-Day "EcoCleanse" Program, as outlined beginning on page 136.

8:00am—Drink 16-ounces of ionized alkaline water *the rainforest way*; feel free to add the juice of one lemon. This will flush your kidneys from a night of cellular shifts and change. Take 6 capsules of probiotics with 2-4 tablespoons of The Alkalizer.

8:30am—Take the "EcoCleanse" Drink.

9:00am—Begin your "EcoJuice" day with a liver/gallbladder cleansing drink. The recipe is 4 large granny smith apples, 1 large unpeeled lemon, 2" piece of fresh ginger, 1 jalapeno or habareno chili pepper and 1 large beet. This juice will not only help to cleanse the stagnant waste and stones from your liver/gallbladder, it will also assist in eliminating any unwanted yeast and parasites.

10:00am—Over the next hour, drink 4-6 ounces of water every 30 minutes. Feel free to add the juice of a lemon or a tablespoon of powdered greens.

Take the "EcoCleanse" Herbs.

11:00am—Juice yourself a powerful kidney-cleansing drink consisting of 8 carrots, 2 unpeeled cucumbers and 1 large beet.

12:00 noon—Over the next hour, drink 4-6 ounces of water every 30 minutes. Feel free to add the juice of a lemon or a tablespoon of powdered greens.

Take the "EcoCleanse" Drink.

1:00pm—Try my *Ultimate Alkalizer!* Juice 6 carrots and one entire bunch of celery. Over the next two hours, drink 4-6 ounces of alternating juice and water every 30 minutes. Feel free to add the juice of a lemon or a tablespoon of powdered greens to your water.

2:00pm— Over the next hour, drink 4-6 ounces of water every 30 minutes. Feel free to add the juice of a lemon or a tablespoon of powdered greens.

Take the "EcoCleanse" Herbs.

3:00pm—Juice yourself another powerful liver/gallbladder cleansing drink. This time, juice 6 carrots, 2 Granny Smith apples, 1 large beet, 6 celery stalks, and 1 unpeeled lemon.

4:00pm—Over the next hour, drink 4-6 ounces of water every 30 minutes. Feel free to add the juice of a lemon or a tablespoon of powdered greens.

Take the "EcoCleanse" Drink.

5:00pm—Enjoy a spicy and filling "Alkalizing-V8" juice for your last drink of the day. Juice 3 carrots, 3 tomatoes, 3 celery stalks, 1 large beet, 1/2 bunch parsley leaves, 4 Romaine lettuce leaves, 4 watercress twigs, and 1 handful spinach. Spice it up with a couple of peeled garlic cloves and 1/2 habanero pepper.

5:30pm—Take the "EcoCleanse" Herbs.

> *Note* If it's cold outside and you'd like to "warm your bones," feel free to enjoy a warm cup of your favorite herbal tea during the day such as chamomile, peppermint, pau d'arco or cardamom found at most health food stores. Extremely high in antioxidants, my favorite tea is "Living Qi Organic Matcha Green Tea" from Japan. This UDSA and IMO (International Maritime Organization) certified organic tea infuses you with energy while relaxing you at the same time. In fact, it has been used as a meditation aid by monks for more than 1,000 years. It's a five-star tea.

The 14-Day "EcoCleanse" Program

While *drinking your way to wellness,* allocate the last 14 days to cleanse all of the accumulated toxins and acid waste out of your entire intestinal tract. Intestinal cleanse supplements that promote the elimination of environmental toxins and acid waste out of the body are more essential today than ever before. Not only have most of us been eating loads of processed chemicalized foods that are "eco-unfriendly" to our body's ecology, the earth's ecology and the environment we live in has become one big chemical "soup pot!" Thus, like periodically changing the oil in your car, cleansing the old toxic waste out of your body before pouring in the new is a major factor in your overall eco-logical and bio-logical success.

Over time, as toxic waste from undigested food particles and environmental toxins builds up in the intestinal tract, in order to protect itself from the acids, the body produces a mucoid plaque lining on the intestinal wall. This plaque inhibits the intake of nutrients and the proper elimination of wastes along with fostering the overgrowth of yeast and unfriendly bacteria.

The following supplemental products are among some of the most effective in the industry in removing the accumulated waste and mucoid plaque out of the intestinal tract.

> *Note* Mucoid plaque is a term coined by Dr. Richard Anderson, a naturopath and researcher, describing an unnatural, harmful coating of a thick, rubbery mucus-like material and food residue, which he states exists in the entire gastrointestinal tracts of almost everyone.

Just be sure to take the time to precleanse so that your body has the electrolyte/minerals and probiotics it needs to do deep cleansing, as this program is not only one of the most effective cleanses on the market, it's the most intense.

> *Note* If you have used or are presently using a different cleanse program than the one I'm suggesting, just be sure that the ingredients are powerful enough to remove mucoid plaque.

The "EcoCleanse" Supplements

The "EcoCleanse" Drink

Psyllium a time-proven fiber used mostly in treating bowel conditions. Naturopaths who specialize in treating bowel conditions will tell you that nothing else is comparable to psyllium husk powder. When purchasing psyllium, it is important to note that psyllium husk powder should not be confused with psyllium seed or whole psyllium husk. If you use the seed or husk version, you'll need at least twice as much as the powder and, when it comes to cleansing the intestines, psyllium seed is practically useless.

Bentonite a hydrated liquid healing clay with a long history of therapeutic use.

Bentonite acts like a sponge, absorbing an amazing amount of toxic debris from the entire alimentary canal. It can absorb 40 times or more its own weight in toxins, bacteria and parasites. Its very important that it has been hydrated, as powdered bentonite has caused severe constipation, pain and in some cases, hospitalization. It should always be used with psyllium husk powder. The combination of bentonite and psyllium works to pull loosened mucoid plaque from the walls of the intestinal tract. The loosened matter then adheres to the bulk of the psyllium, allowing a quick exit from the body.

> *Note* These two products make up your "EcoCleanse" drink. Synergistically, they work together to quickly draw the toxins out of your body that are being released by the "EcoCleanse" herbs. If you don't like the taste, simply add a small amount of organic apple juice. If this doesn't work, feel free to try the 14-day "EcoCleanse" without the "EcoCleanse" drink. Because I now eat a mostly raw food diet and my body is fairly clean, I don't always take the "EcoCleanse" drink. Therefore, whenever I do a 21-Day (or even a 40-Day) "EcoJuice" cleanse once or twice a year, I only use the two intestinal herbal products for the entire 21 days. But you need to be the judge because no one knows your body and your level of readiness like you!

The "EcoCleanse" Herbs

Herbal Intestinal Cleanse an herbal formula as previously described on page 132. These herbs help to soften and break up toxic waste material while detoxifying cells. An herbal combination that works well for this includes plantain, cascara sagrada, barberry, peppermint, sheep sorrel, fennel seed, ginger root, myrrh gum, red raspberry, rhubarb root, goldenseal, and lobelia. This herbal formula, along with herbal intestinal nutrition, prepares the mucoid plaque for removal and neutralizes stored intestinal toxins such as pesticides, drugs, pathogenic microorganisms and even some parasites. When this plaque is removed, the lymphatic drainage points open, which in turn allows the toxins and sludge to be dumped from all areas of the body. It also helps to cleanse the liver, skin, lungs, kidneys along with other body tissues. In addition, it allows the 22 enzymes secreted by the intestines to reach the food we eat and complete the digestive processes and assists the absorption of nutrients.

Herbal Intestinal Nutrition an herbal formula that has been found to be an exceptional balanced nutritional supplement to support the body before, during and after cleansing. It works synergistically with the Herbal Intestinal Cleanse formula and, in addition, it helps to strengthen all of the organs, especially the heart, kidneys, liver, gall bladder, skin and lymphatic system. It helps strengthen the body so it can be more effective in the elimination process and help reduce the possibility of toxic overloads. Five of these herbs were in the diet of Dr. Anderson when he was living in the mountains on only raw, fresh herbs and discovered the magical formula that removed mucoid plaque like nothing else could. This second formula included: alfalfa leaf, chickweed, dandelion root, hawthorne berry, Irish moss, kelp, licorice, marshmallow root, rose hips, shavegrass, and yellow dock.

Note These two herbal formulas work together to help remove toxins from all areas of the body as well as the mucoid plaque. Just be prepared to see some amazing things coming out of you. Start on the lowest recommended amount. If you're not experiencing any detox reactions, keep increasing until you've reached the highest recommended amount. Just remember that everyone is different and the amounts will always vary between people. Learn to listen and work with your body.

The Directions

The "EcoCleanse" Drink

Psyllium
2 teaspoons 3-5 times a day on an empty stomach mixed with liquid bentonite.

Liquid Bentonite
1 tablespoon 3-5 times a day on an empty stomach mixed with psyllium. Place psyllium and bentonite in a shaker bottle with 12 ounces of water; then shake and drink right away.

The "EcoCleanse" Herbs

Herbal Intestinal Cleanse
4-6 capsules 3-5 times a day on an empty stomach.

Herbal Intestinal Nutrition
4-6 capsules 3-5 times a day on an empty stomach.

The "EcoCleanse" Schedule

Begin the 14-Day "EcoCleanse" during the second week of the 21-day *drink your way to wellness* program. The results of this cleansing program are dramatically enhanced when taking a daily colonic (colon irrigation) every day during days 7-14 of your cleanse. The "open system" colonic machine is my favorite because it's a more natural process, but a "closed system" is also very effective.

Days 1-7

Begin the first seven days of the "EcoCleanse" during week two of the 21-day *drink your way to wellness* program while enjoying all the freshly-prepared "EcoJuice" and ionized alkaline water you desire. Continue taking your prebiotics and probiotics.

Under 150 lbs.

> 8:30am – "EcoCleanse" Drink
> 10:00am – "EcoCleanse" Herbs
> 12noon – "EcoCleanse" Drink
> 2:00am – "EcoCleanse" Herbs
> 4:00pm – "EcoCleanse" Drink
> 5:30pm – "EcoCleanse" Herbs

Over 150 lbs.

> 7:00pm – "EcoCleanse" Drink
> 8:30pm – "EcoCleanse" Herbs

If your weight is under 150 lbs., take each 3 times per day – 1 ½ hours apart.
If your weight is over 150 lbs., take each 4 times per day – 1 ½ hours apart.

Days 7-14

Begin the second seven days of the "EcoCleanse" during week three of the 21-day *drink your way to wellness* program. During this phase, drink nothing but water for the last 7 days of the program. Be sure to drink approximately one gallon of ionized alkaline water every day. Lots of water is essential to the success of the intestinal cleanse program.

For a less intense cleanse, feel free to add a small amount of freshly-prepared apple juice to your cleansing drink. Continue taking the prebiotics and probiotics.

And again, if you're already *clean and green* inside, the "EcoCleanse" drink is optional.

Under 150 lbs.

    7:00am – "EcoCleanse" Drink
    8:30am – "EcoCleanse" Herbs
  10:00am – "EcoCleanse" Drink
  11:30am – "EcoCleanse" Herbs
    1:00pm – "EcoCleanse" Drink
    2:30pm – "EcoCleanse" Herbs
    4:00pm – "EcoCleanse" Drink
    5:30pm – "EcoCleanse" Herbs

Over 150 lbs.

    7:00pm – "EcoCleanse" Drink
    8:30pm – "EcoCleanse" Herbs

If your weight is under 150 lbs., take each 4 times per day – 1 ½ hours apart.
If your weight is over 150 lbs., take each 5 times per day – 1 ½ hours apart.

Additional Detox & Restoration Therapies

• Sunlight—Spend an hour a day in the early morning or late afternoon sun.

• Deep Breathing—Spend 30 minutes every day focused on your breath and doing some repetitive deep-breathing exercises as outlined in Chapter 7. Your lungs are an elimination organ and will greatly assist you in removing acids.

• Colon hydrotherapy—Take one colonic a day during the last 7 days of your intestinal cleanse.

• Skin brushing— The skin is our body's largest eliminative organ. Brushing your skin with a skin brush once or twice a day helps the lymphatic system to cleanse itself of excess toxins that have collected in your lymph glands.

- Detox baths—Soak in Celtic Crystal Bath Salts for 20 minutes 3 times a week during your cleanse. Feel free to add 1 cup apple cider vinegar and 1/4 cup ground ginger and/or your favorite essential oil. Detox baths also help to eliminate toxins out of the skin.

- Alternating hot and cold baths—Take one a day for 20-30 minutes during your fast.

- Infrared sauna—Take one a day for 20-30 minutes during your fast.

- Rebounding—Bouncing and breathing exercises at least 20 minutes every day on a mini-trampoline is an excellent way to flush the lymphatic system of toxic waste and oxygenate the body.

- Yoga, Qigong, Walking—Not so strenuous, meditative forms of exercise during your fast are extremely beneficial.

- Massage—Treat yourself to a massage several times a week.

- Forgiveness and emotional release work—As your body releases the old, accumulated toxic waste, old emotional issues and thoughts can come up to be released. Acid thoughts and feelings can also create an acidic environment. But if you learn a process of true forgiveness, that of letting go of false perceptions and old realities while cleansing your body, you will not only cleanse your body but your soul, as well.

Breaking Your Fast

Breaking your 21-day "EcoJuice" fast and "EcoCleanse" is almost as important as the fasting cleanse itself, so do it wisely. Day 1-3, consume a diet of raw fruits in season to keep the cleansing process going, and continue to drink as much freshly-prepared vegetable juice and ionized alkaline water as you'd like. Then, over the next few days, begin to incorporate the *EcoDiet* food program: Level One or Level Two as outlined on page 150. Along with your daily food program, I also recommend the following daily supplement program.

Daily Supplement Program

Continue taking the "EcoCleanse" herbs 2-3 times a day between meals along with the probiotics and prebiotics for 3-6 months. Be sure to also drink lots of ionized alkaline water *the rainforest way*. If you do, over time, your intestinal ecology will not only be thoroughly cleansed, it will be restored to normal function. You'll also want to continue taking digestive enzymes with every meal, as they will assist in proper digestion.

STEP #3: THE "GET CLEAN" CANDIDA CLEANSE

This final *Get Clean* step is for those of you who have an overgrowth of Candida; some of you know that you do and others, don't. Just know that if you've tried every cleanse (including the one I'm suggesting), or weight loss program on the market and end up failing because of food cravings (especially sugar), your body is most likely overridden with Candida. And no matter how strong your will power, these cravings are in control. They'll march you right over to the refrigerator only hours after deciding to *drink your way to wellness* and before you know it, you're opening the freezer door to get an ice cream fix. I know because I've been there.

Even though I considered myself to be a vegan-vegetarian because I didn't eat meat or dairy, I was really a junkitarian who was addicted to the health food store version of sugary junk foods. This is because my bloodstream and intestines were overrun with "yeasty-beasties" and didn't even know it. I craved everything from rice and soy ice cream and desserts, vegan chocolate-chocolate chip cookies, organic chips, pizza, pasta, bread, organic wine, veggie subs, and so on. I really wanted to change, but couldn't. These "yeasty-beasties" were in control and my belly was blowing up like a "Pillsbury Dough Boy." Yeast have a mind of their own and they send out their own SOS signal, signaling you to feed them and feed them now!

It has been estimated that 80% of Americans have, or have had, a yeast or Candida infection. While those numbers are staggering, most people are unaware that Candida overgrowth could be at the root of their ecological breakdown. If left unchecked, Candida can cause a plethora of health challenges to arise.

These health challenges can show up as incapacitating fatigue, lack of concentration, alcoholism, mental confusion, insomnia, nervousness, hyperactivity, agitation, short term memory loss, phobias, persistent drowsiness, clinical depression, headaches, muscle and joint pain, mood swings, dizziness, lack of coordination, ear sensitivity/ringing/itching or fluid in the ears, mucous in stools, postnasal drip, frequent colds, recurring strep throat, sinusitis, bronchitis, heartburn/acid reflux, nervous irritability, tightness of the chest, white stuff in the throat, coated tongue, dark circles under the eyes, bad breath, thyroid problems, chronic dental problems, blood sugar disorders, and the list goes on.

With this program, you don't have to change your diet...it will change on its own!

More severe problems that are often accompanied by Candida overgrowth are irritable bowel syndrome, leaky gut, Crohn's disease, Celiac disease, autism, ADD, ADHD, fibromyalgia, cancer, diabetes, hypoglycemia, chronic fatigue, Epstein-Barr virus, pneumonia, lupus, hiatal hernia, and hormone imbalances. In fact, from all of my research, I have concluded that Candida overgrowth, which is almost never diagnosed, may be at the root of most every disease known.

The great news is, with this program, every sugar craving you've ever had will disappear once and for all and mostly, without any effort. No will power is needed because you'll be getting to the root of why you overeat and crave foods you know aren't good for you. However, in the beginning, you may have to do this program several times to reach the success you desire.

The problem is that yeast thrives on sugar, and so does your brain. Unfortunately, it's the yeast in your intestines that gets first dibs on almost any type of sugar you eat. Meanwhile, your brain cells scream at you to eat more because they didn't get their fair share, so you eat and eat and eat then balloon up, your weight soars out of control and your self-image goes down the toilet.

There are several causes of Candida overgrowth:

First is diet. Remember that Candida eats blood sugar and if the food supply becomes excessive, Candida multiplies to keep up with the excessive food demand. If a person's insulin is unable to escort the sugar out of the bloodstream, the sugar can't get out and Candida keeps blooming. And what keeps the insulin from escorting sugar out is the over consumption of fat—the more fat (especially saturated and trans fat) in your diet, the less effective insulin is at getting sugar out of the blood stream. Keep your fat intake between 10-15%.

Second is drugs. Prescribed medications such as antibiotics, vaccinations, birth control pills, and steroids disturbs the balance of the friendly bacteria in the intestines and allows yeast (Candida) to go out of control. This is why women often get a vaginal yeast infection after taking antibiotics.

Third is chemicals. Chemicals such as pesticides, aspartame, MSG, chlorinated water, preservatives, or even the toxic metals in your mouth like mercury fillings can cause yeast to grow out of control.

Fourth is inorganic calcium. Some researchers report that Candida also overgrows due to a deficiency of ionic calcium. Dr. Norman Walker in his book *Fruit and Vegetable Juice* states that cooking calcium-containing foods (like pasteurized dairy products) renders calcium inorganic which in turns clogs up the organs, joints and tissues. He advocates foods high in organic sodium such as celery and zucchini to balance the pH that cause the yeast to grow out of control, and help remove the pile-up of inorganic calcium.

How To Test Yourself For Candida

Fortunately, there's a simple saliva test to determine if your underlying health or weight problem might just be coming from an overgrowth of Candida.

First thing in the morning, get a clear glass and fill it with warm water. Rinse out your mouth, then work up some saliva and spit into the glass of water. Keep an eye on the water every few minutes for up to one hour, especially the first few minutes. If you have a Candida infection, you'll see one of three, or even all three of the following:

1. Strings traveling down into the water from the saliva floating on top.

2. Nasty looking saliva at the bottom of the glass.

3. Cloudy specks suspended in the water.

This test is more accurate first thing in the morning because Candida concentrates in saliva overnight. The more you see of any or all of these and the faster you see it, the worse the overgrowth. If you spit and almost immediately see stuff falling out of the saliva, know that you have it bad. If 20 minutes after spitting you see just a little bit falling out of the saliva, you have it, but not as extensive. If the saliva just floats on top, and the water stays perfectly clear, you probably don't have Candida overgrowth.

Unfortunately, once you have an overgrowth of Candida, it won't leave on its own. Candida cells are very stubborn and you must do whatever it takes to eliminate excess Candida, restore your intestinal ecology and prevent Candida from proliferating any further. I have found that it takes approximately 60 days to completely eradicate Candida overgrowth. Just remember to be patient…it does take time.

> **Note** For best results, complete the 14-day intestinal "EcoCleanse" before doing the Candida Cleanse. If, however, you are suffering from food cravings, feel free to start the Candida cleanse at the beginning of the *drink your way to wellness program* and during the 14-day "EcoCleanse."

Candida Cleanse Supplements

Probiotics a formula designed to provide selected beneficial microflora to the intestinal tract for the purpose of replenishing needed friendly flora and eradicating the overgrowth of Candida. Candida is one member of a community of microorganisms that lives within the ecology of the intestinal tract in balance with beneficial bacteria. In a healthy intestinal tract, normal populations of friendly bacteria keep Candida in check. A healthy intestinal tract should contain approximately 85% alkaline-producing friendly bacteria such as bifidobacterium and 15% acid-producing bacteria such as Lactobacillus acidophilus. Under normal conditions only a small number of Candida organisms live in the intestines. Under abnormal conditions, however, a large number of Candida and other potentially harmful organisms exist: 15% friendly bacteria and 85% harmful. To remedy this, look for a powerful probiotic formulation that contains beneficial microflora, such as L. acidophilus DDS-1, E. faecium, L. casei, L. bulgaricus, L. plantarum and L. salivarius.

Oxygen a product that highly oxygenates every cell of the body. And, as you now know by now, viruses, amoebas, parasites, fungi or bacteria cannot live in a highly oxygenated environment. Every cell of the body needs oxygen to function properly because oxygen is essential to cleansing as well as feeding your cells. To accomplish this, your cells must be bathed in the right kind of water: a form that is both highly oxygenated and is usable to the body. Thus, a stabilized oxygen product added to 4-6 ounces of ionized alkaline water several times a day is needed to help accomplish this very important goal. Coupled with a highly alkalizing pH formula that contains cesium chloride, rubidium chloride and potassium, a state of wellbeing is almost always guaranteed. Magnesium oxide powders are the most effective.

Systemic Enzymes a highly active formula that contain enzymes which split proteins into shorter chains of amino acids, thus providing multiple health benefits, in particular, anti-inflammatory, anti-fibrotic and blood-purifying effects. Systemic enzymes contain high levels of protease, amylase, lipase, serrapeptase, bromelain, papain, cellulase, along with other active enzymes, needed to break down any stored undigested fats, carbohydrates and proteins that yeast and parasites feed on. Systemic enzyme therapy has long been one of the master keys holistic physicians worldwide have used to turn almost every degenerative problem around. When taken in therapeutic doses and taken just before and in between meals, enzymes serve as one of the greatest tools to assist you on your way back to a state of health and wellbeing.

Organic Colloidal Silver a laboratory produced, crystal clear and virtually tasteless product made from 99.99% pure silver hydrosols and ultra-pure medical-grade water that is highly effective against most pathogenic organisms known, including viruses, bacteria, and Candida. The actively charged particle size of 0.0008 microns (validated by Transmission Electron Microscopy) and ultra-fine dispersion greatly enhances the bioavailability of these unique silver ions. When theses ultra-small silver particles come in contact with pathogenic organisms, it appears to shut off the pathogen's ability to metabolize oxygen so the pathogen suffocates and dies, generally in 4-6 minutes. In a group of FDA-certified laboratory tests, this type of ultra-small silver topically killed 7.85 billion cells of Candida at a rate of 99.99% in 60 minutes with only three drops. If you do have an overgrowth of Candida, you'll also want to add Aloe Vera juice every day to transport the silver into the intestinal tract.

Grapefruit Seed Extract an extract made by first converting grapefruit seeds and pulp into a liquid that is loaded with compounds shown to be very effective in eliminating various types of internal and external infections caused from parasites, viruses, bacteria, fungi and more. It is known to naturally detoxify, enhance and support the immune system while alkalizing the blood. Alkalizing the body's fluids is one of the single most important health regeneration benefits available, as disease-causing microforms such as fungus, bacteria, virus, etc., cannot survive in an alkaline oxygenated environment.

The Directions

Probiotics
Take 6 capsules on an empty stomach with *The Alkalizer* first thing in the morning for one month then 3 capsules thereafter for 3 months.

Oxygen
If using a liquid, take 1 dropper 3 times a day on an empty stomach; work up to 2 droppers 3 times a day. If using a magnesium oxide powder, take 1-2 teaspoons 2-3 times a day on an empty stomach.

Systemic Enzymes
Take 6-12 capsules between meals 3 times a day on an empty stomach.

Organic Colloidal Silver
Mix 2 tablespoons organic colloidal silver with 2 tablespoons aloe vera juice and drink 3 times a day on an empty stomach. To avoid detox reactions, begin with 1 tablespoon each for a few days then increase accordingly. While taking

this silver, take 3 probiotics before bedtime to make sure your friendly bacteria balance stays intact.

Grapefruit Seed Extract

Mix 20 drops in 4-8 ounces of water 3 times a day on an empty stomach. To avoid detox reactions, begin with 7 drops then increase accordingly.

Candida Diet   a low carbohydrate diet can be helpful in the beginning (but not a requirement) for those who have Candida, even though the *Get Clean Go Green EcoDiet* is a low fat, high carbohydrate diet. This means that for 60-90 days, after the *drink your way to wellness* program, you'll want to avoid high-glycemic fruits such as bananas, mangoes and watermelon; natural sugars such as raw honey; starchy foods such as pasta, potatoes and bread; and fermented foods such as apple cider vinegar, miso, cheese, and sauerkraut. And absolutely no alcohol.

Low-glycemic fruits such as green apples, black cherries, berries, pears, grapefruit, plums, peaches and grapes are acceptable in very small amounts, especially when eaten in season and when mixed in a green smoothie. Whenever you have a salad, avoid most store-bought salad dressings. Simply toss your salad with a small amount of olive, hemp or flax oil, lemon juice, garlic, minced ginger and your favorite culinary herbs. Some people have even found that they need to follow an all green, no fruit (with the exception of lemon, limes, grapefruit and berries), grains or beans in order to eradicate Candida, especially if the infection has been long-standing. Either way, after 90 days, your internal environment should be back in balance at which time a more ecologically-balanced diet can be consumed...an *EcoDiet* that supports a healthy ecology.

Just keep in mind that Candida consumes blood sugar and when there is too much sugar in your bloodstream, Candida multiplies to keep up with the excessive food demand. If your insulin is unable to escort the sugar out of the bloodstream, the sugar can't get out and Candida keeps blooming. What keeps the insulin from escorting sugar out is the over consumption of fat—the more fat in your diet the less effective insulin is at getting sugar out of the blood stream. Thus, our total caloric daily intake of fat should never exceed 15%.

A healthy formula is: the more fruit you eat, the less fat you should eat—the less fruit you eat, the more fat you can eat.

Now take a moment and image with me a food program powerful enough to enliven your body's ecology in a way that prevents most ecological breakdowns while heightening your overall sense of wellbeing. Well, I believe, the *Get Clean Go Green* Program is powerful enough to do just that! Just remember that when the Candida overgrowth subsides…your food cravings will subside at the same time.

In other words,

You won't have to change your diet, it will change on its own!

PART TWO

THE "GO GREEN" PROGRAM

Like the grade of gasoline we burn in our car's engine affects the outer environment in a positive or negative way, the grade of food we burn in our body's engine affects our internal environment in a positive or negative way. Gasoline is classified by three grades: regular, midgrade and premium. Likewise, food can be classified by three grades: regular, midgrade and premium.

Regular has no classification. This diet is the SAD (Standard American Diet).

Midgrade is classified as Level One.

Premium is classified as Level Two.

Level One consists of a plant-based organic *whole foods diet*, which places emphasis on vegetables, fruits, whole grains, beans, nuts and seeds. This diet is not only animal-free, it is dairy-free, low in fat and high in fiber. On this plan, you would follow the 80/20 acid-alkaline food principle: 80% alkaline foods and 20% mild acid foods. You would follow the *seasons of change*…a 100% raw food diet in the summer with lots of seasonal fruits and almost no fat; a less raw food diet in the autumn and winter with lots of vegetables, grains and beans as your foundation and a little more fat (not to exceed 15% total caloric intake); then in the spring, you would reduce your fat intake to 10% and enjoy lots of greens and sprouts.

Level Two consists of a plant-based organic *raw foods diet*, which places emphasis on vegetables, fruits, sprouted beans and/or cultured nuts and seeds. This diet is also animal and dairy-free, low in fat and high in fiber. On this plan, you would also follow the acid-alkaline food principle: 80% alkaline foods and 20% mild acid foods. The difference between Level One and Level Two is that everything is always eaten in its raw, living state.

An important principle to always keep in mind with both Level One and Level Two is to always adjust your diet according to each changing season; i.e., in the summertime, fruits are in season so eat lots of them and hardly any fat. During the wintertime (unless you live in the Bahamas!!), most fruits are not in season so eat more fat and greens and hardly any fruit. Thus, if you simply use "seasonal sense" and follow

---

"Just as food causes chronic disease, it can be the most powerful cure."
– Hippocrates, the Father of Medicine

---

nature's laws and not man's (including mine), you'll win every time!! I'm simply setting an acid-alkaline *EcoDiet* guideline for you to follow.

The good news is that you don't even need *specific foods* for *specific problems*. An overall healthy *EcoDiet* eaten over time is your key to success. Let your diet be a lifestyle and not something you go on today and off tomorrow. Thus, all you have to do is to stop acidifying your internal environment with extremely acid-forming foods and start alkalizing!

So what does it mean to Go Green?

Go Green means to burn the right types of food for fuel within your internal environment; a way of eating that honors your body as the earth and the earth as yourself.

Level One: The 80/20 Plan
80% Alkaline Foods – 20% Acid Foods

The Level One 80/20 plan is classified as the four-star environmentally sustainable "midgrade fuel" way of eating, which will greatly assist you in your *go green* alkalizing process. It will also assist you in shifting from an animal-based junkitarian diet to a plant-based whole foods diet, and without much effort. This program is designed to do three things: (1) to keep your storehouse full of alkaline minerals and enzymes, (2) to replenish and maintain your storehouse if your alkaline reserves and enzymes are low or already bankrupt and (3) to keep your cells so nutritionally saturated that your cravings for acid-forming junk foods will steadily diminish, without much effort.

The plan consists of a daily consumption of 80% mild and strong alkaline-forming foods and 20% mild acid-forming foods. To be more specific, your Level One "Go Green" *EcoDiet* menu would look like this:

80% Alkaline Food & Drink
40% strong alkaline-forming foods
40% mild alkaline-forming foods
These foods are best eaten in their raw, living state.

20% Acid Food & Drink
20% mild acid-forming foods
These foods can be eaten slightly cooked.

To help with a clearer understanding of what this would look like, imagine looking at a plate of food you're about to eat for breakfast, lunch or dinner. Simply put, at least 80% of the foods you see on your plate would be foods from the alkaline-forming list and up to 20% would be foods from the mild acid-forming food list: 80% of your daily fare would be eaten fresh and raw—20% would be eaten lightly grilled, baked or steamed.

For example, the food on your plate would consist of organic whole grain sprouted pasta with pesto and a large green leafy salad. The sprouted pasta (made by Ezekiel) would take up no more than 20% of the food space on your plate while the other 80% would be a large green leafy salad and maybe a small amount of streamed vegetables. It's very simple. All you need to do is to become familiar with which foods are alkaline-forming, and which ones are acid-forming. The rule of thumb is to remember that leafy greens are the most alkalizing foods; all other vegetables are second; fruits are third; and grains, beans, nuts and seeds are fourth. Remember to soak your grains, beans, nuts and seeds for 24 hours before consuming.

Sprouted Grains, Beans, Nuts & Seeds
Fruits
Vegetables
Leafy Greens

"GO GREEN" SUPREME SUPERFOODS

Another group of "Go Green" *EcoDiet* foods for both Level One and Level Two are *Superfoods*. Superfood is a term to describe a particular food that has a high phytonutrient content that may offer tremendous health benefits as a result; and remember, phytonutrients are nutrients derived from plants that form a part of a plant's immune system, protecting them from disease, injury, extreme weather conditions and more, and have shown to be necessary for sustaining human life.

The Oxford English Dictionary includes citations for superfood in the general sense of "a food considered especially nutritious or otherwise beneficial to health and wellbeing," dating from 1915 and 1949, as well as more recent examples. These multitasking powerful superfoods are high in antioxidants and various nutrients proven to prevent and, in some cases, reverse the effects of aging and disease. Superfoods are so nutrient-dense that they also help to eliminate food cravings.

According to various health experts, the top 10 health-promoting superfoods include berries, kiwi, broccoli, tomatoes, sea vegetables, quinoa, beans, hot peppers, nuts and seeds. While these top 10 serve us well, there's a new category of superfoods that I call, *Supreme Superfoods*. Supreme Superfoods are foods that most have never heard of. But studies have shown that the following top 10 *Supreme Superfoods* are the most nutritious and powerful foods in the world. Added to a morning smoothie, or made into a morning *Supreme Superfood Shot*, these foods will fuel your cell's engine for peak performance.

Green Powders a nutrient-rich organic green powder that includes various young cereal grasses such as wheatgrass and barley grass, as well as vegetable powder concentrates. Green powder's high alkalinity assists in the elimination of acids, weight loss, alleviating chronic fatigue symptoms, strengthening your immunity, improving mental acuity and cleansing every cell of your body. Nutritionally, green powders are close cousins to dark green leafy vegetables, but offer far greater levels of "nutrient density." An ounce of these concentrated green foods contains more health-promoting phytonutrients than found in an ounce of green vegetables. The results of many experimental studies show that green foods have marked beneficial effects on cholesterol, blood pressure, immune response and cancer prevention. These effects are attributed, in part, to their high concentrations of chlorophyll, which is the phytochemical that gives green-leafy plants their green hue. Like green plants oxygenate our planet's atmosphere, they also oxygenate our body's atmosphere.

Superfood Berries are phytonutrient-rich berries such as goji, acai and camu camu. These berries are extremely high in dietary fiber, rich in fatty acids and are loaded with antioxidants. In addition, berries contain high levels of the healthy monounsaturated fatty acid oleic acid, omega 6, vitamin A and calcium. Due to the highly perishable nature of the raw fruit, these berries, other than goji, are only available in powder form, which make a wonderful super-charged addition to your morning smoothies.

Nuts are powerful antioxidant and anti-inflammatory superfoods. Studies involving more than 220,000 people show that diets that include nuts help reduce the risk of heart disease, the leading killer of both men and women in the United States. As an example, the famous Seventh Day Adventists study followed the diets of more than 30,000 church members over a 12-year period. The results showed that, even in this healthy-living, largely vegetarian group, those who ate nuts at least five times per week cut their risk of dying from coronary heart disease by 48 percent, compared with those who ate nuts less than once weekly. They also cut their risk of a non-fatal heart attack by 51 percent.

Seeds are phytonutrient-rich superfoods. Seeds such as milk thistle, flax, chia, pumpkin, hemp, sunflower, and sesame are high in fiber, vitamin E and monoun-saturated fats, are known to keep our hearts healthy and our body disease free. These health-promoting seeds are also great sources of protein, minerals, zinc and other life-enhancing nutrients. Numerous studies have also shown that these seeds can actually prevent weight gain, the development of heart disease and the accumulation of LDL cholesterol.

Sprouts are amongst one of the top health-promoting superfoods. One of their many health benefits is the sprouting biochemistry that transforms the seed into a plant, a process that unlocks the resources stored in seeds so as to become more bio-available to the growing sprout. Clover sprouts contain the most significant dietary sources of isoflavones of any sprout variety. Isoflavone is a plant flavonoid with the capacity to act as an antioxidant with anti-cancer properties, according to researchers. Clover sprout's dark green leaves have an abundance of chlorophyll and blood cleansing properties. The China Study, performed by Professor T. Campbell and son, outlines the positive effects on cancer sufferers by using plant proteins from sprouts. They found that two day old mung bean sprouts (when the radicle and hypocotyl have just emerged) have approximately 23% protein along with other vital nutrients needed by cancer patients.

Rice Bran Complex a phytonutrient-dense complex now hailed as the new superfood. Rice bran contains a quite amazing number of nutrients. Rice bran complex contains just about all the vitamins you would ever need. Rice bran contains phytosterols, polysaccharides, beta-sitosterol, fiber, Vitamin E complex and a large complement of B vitamins; these even include B15, a vital antioxidant. Rice bran complex also boasts co-enzyme Q10, omega 3 and 6 fatty acids and even oleic acid also found in olive oil. Try adding a scoop or two to your daily diet; you'll be glad you did!

Maca Root Powder is considered by top researchers to be a true adaptogen (a natural herb product that is proposed to increase the body's resistance to stress, trauma, anxiety and fatigue) and aggressively touted as the "superfood of the Andes" by the natural products industry. Working in tandem with the body's natural rhythms, maca root helps rebuild weak immune systems, balance hormones, re-mineralize poorly nourished bodies, and increase energy and endurance. Each maca root contains over 55 naturally occurring, beneficial phytochemicals. These naturally occurring chemicals include important hormonal precursors and sterols proven time and time again to assist the human body in a number of recognizable ways. Most people feel their mood and energy level lift in an instant.

Bee Pollen is one of nature's most powerful superfoods. The early Egyptian and early Chinese civilizations both have used it as a cure-all medicine for thousands of years. In fact, the Greek physician Hippocrates, recognized as the father of modern medicine, used bee pollen as a healing substance over 2,500 years ago. Today natural health care practitioners often refer to bee pollen as an herbal "fountain of youth" that can be used for everything from weight loss to cancer prevention.

Royal Jelly is a superfood that has also been revered as a "fountain of youth" since the dawn of history. The healing power and health benefits of royal jelly are still one of the most sought-after subjects in modern times. It is hailed as the crown jewel among beehive products. A rich, creamy white opalescent liquid, royal jelly is produced by worker bees and used exclusively for the nourishment of the queen bee, who is recognized for her longevity (compared with regular worker bees–several years vs. just 1-2 months), energy, and stamina for reproductive capability. Royal jelly is extremely high in nutritional value and is popular as a skin rejuvenator. Royal jelly is high in proteins, rich in natural hormones and rich in amino acids.

UMF® Active Manuka Honey is considered a healing honey. Collected from a plant that is unique to New Zealand, *UMF®* Active Manuka honey is highly acclaimed for its medicinal properties. Manuka flowers appear in the spring and are much loved by the honeybees. This honey is considered healing honey through scientifically-based laboratory studies. It was found to have high levels of hydrogen peroxide, which has immune-enhancing and antibacterial properties known as UMF®, the same substance used by white blood cells to neutralize unfriendly bacteria. The active UMF® component of Manuka honey is rated between 5+ and 25+. Manuka Honey USA has found that the best rating for internal use is 16+ to 19+. (UMF is the name of a very beneficial bacteria found in some strains of manuka honey, but not in all. So be sure that the honey you purchase has a UMF rating.)

The Directions

Supreme Superfood Green Powder
Take 1-2 tablespoons a day in juice or water.

Superfood Berries or Powder
Take 2-3 tablespoons a day in your smoothie.

Nuts
Eat a small handful every day.

Seeds
Grind a variety into a powder and have a tablespoon a day in water or smoothie.

Sprouts
Eat or juice as many as you desire every day.

Rice Bran Complex
Take 3-8 tablespoons a day in juice or water.

Maca Root Powder
Take 1-2 tablespoons a day in juice or water.

Bee Pollen
Take 1-2 tablespoons a day.

Royal Jelly
Enjoy 1 tablespoon a day.

UMF® Active Manuka Honey
Enjoy 1-2 tablespoons a day in lemon water.

First thing in the morning, try my organic triple *Supreme Superfood Shot*. It's definitely a high-octane way to start the day!

Supreme Superfood Shot

1/4 cup goji berries
1 tablespoon acai berry powder
1/2 cup raw noni or goji berry juice
1 tablespoon active manuka honey
1/2 cup ionized alkaline water
Place in blender and blend until smooth.

To show you how really simple it is to follow the Level One 80/20 Plan, here's a sample week of menu ideas:

A Sample Week

Breakfast Fresh fruit salad in season. Choose from any fruit salad or phytonutrient-rich smoothie in the recipe section or create your own. Feel free to add 1/2 cup cultured nuts or seeds (recipe on page 217) to any breakfast meal or smoothie. In the summer, when fruit is seasonally plentiful, I simply enjoy eating one type of fruit at a time, such as a big bowl of mangoes or a huge piece of watermelon.

- Enjoy a bowl of mangoes or papayas, grapes or some watermelon, whichever fruit is in season.

- Make a Superfood Smoothie—create a delicious phytonutrient-rich smoothie with 2-3 different fruits such as a whole apple, banana and orange along with a 2-3 cups of water. Go ahead...blend the whole fruit, seeds and all. Feel free to add some *Supreme Superfoods* such as acai powder or goji berries.

- Try a Berry Blend—blend 1/2 cup fresh organic raspberries, blueberries, strawberries and blackberries with 2-3 cups of water; add a frozen banana and a green powder blend. Go ahead…be creative!

- Take yourself to the tropics with a Tropical Treat—blend 1/2 cup fresh organic pineapple, mango and papaya with lots of fresh young coconut water or cultured coconut water. Add a banana, 1/2 cup cultured almonds and 2 tablespoons rice bran complex.

- Have a Green Smoothie—blend 1 bunch of stemmed dinosaur kale with your choice of fresh organic fruit, such as mango, banana, pineapple and/or orange with 24 ounces water. Add a tablespoon of your favorite green powder blend.

- Start your day with one of my favorites—juice 2 apples, 1 unpeeled lemon, 1 2-inch piece of ginger, 2 ounces wheatgrass juice; then take it up a "hot notch" with 1/2 habanero pepper.

Lunch Try a large leafy green salad with your favorite pre-soaked grains, beans, nuts or seeds. Choose any salad in the recipe section you wish or again, create your own. When eating pasta, be sure to choose "sprouted" pasta by Ezekiel.

- Organic sprouted brown rice pasta tossed with olive oil, crushed garlic, salt to taste, freshly-chopped basil and lots of cherry tomatoes cut in half, all served on a bed of olive oil and garlic with tossed Arugula.

- Cannellini beans, spiced with cayenne pepper, garlic and Nama Shoyu Unpasteurized Soy Sauce; add strips of roasted red bell peppers and toss. Serve on a warm sprouted tortilla and top with lots of mixed spring greens tossed with olive oil, garlic and salt.

- Organic sprouted brown rice pasta with lots of pesto served with a large green leafy salad.

- A bowl of your favorite organic heirloom grains tossed with steamed veggies and a large green salad on the side.

- A large Caesar salad with a side of sprouted or cooked organic grains.

- An organic baked potato topped with steamed vegetables tossed with lots of olive oil and pressed garlic.

- Mixed green salad tossed with raw or lightly steamed Brussels sprouts, broccoli and cauliflower, sprouted nuts and seeds.

Dinner Eating a lighter fare for dinner such as soup and salad is the healthiest way to end the day. Low in calories, filling up on fiber and water-rich soup and salad also prevents you from overdoing a more high-calorie nighttime fare. Research from Penn

State University shows that eating a first-course salad helps to reduce overall calorie intake at a meal by up to 12%. A study in *Appetite* magazine (November 2007 edition) reported that people who started a meal with vegetable soup ended up eating 20% less than those who skipped the soup. What I've discovered for myself is that when I have soup and salad for dinner, I feel so satisfied that I no longer have late night cravings. Try it for a few weeks and see for yourself.

Here are a few examples that can be found in the Level One & Two recipe section of this book.

- Cream of corn soup served with a kale-avocado salad.
- Lima bean-spinach soup served with a small, chopped veggie salad.
- Split pea soup served with a frieze-radicchio salad tossed in lemon juice and olive oil vinaigrette.
- Miso soup with a yin-yang salad.
- Spinach and sun-dried tomato salad with tomato-basil soup.
- Black bean soup served with a simple side salad made with chopped romaine.
- Lettuce, avocado, tomato, red onion and a dash of Nama Shoyu Unpasteurized Soy Sauce.
- Rosemary-potato soup served with a rainbow salad and miso-good dressing.

Level Two: The 80/20 Raw, Living Food Plan
80% Raw Alkaline Foods – 20% Raw Acid Foods

The Raw Food 80/20 Level Two plan is classified as the five-star environmentally sustainable "premium fuel" way of eating, which will greatly assist you in your *go green* alkalizing process.

This program is also designed to do three things: (1) to keep your storehouse full of alkaline minerals and enzymes, (2) to replenish your storehouse if your alkaline reserves and enzymes are low or already bankrupt and (3) to keep your cells so nutritionally saturated that your cravings for acid-forming foods will steadily diminish, without effort. This plan gives your cellular engine even greater horsepower than the four-star environmentally sustainable way of eating.

The plan consists of a daily consumption of 80% fruits and vegetables, 10% sprouted beans and grains and 10% fat. To be more specific, your EcoDiet menu would look like this:

80% Fruits & Vegetables
40% fruits
40% vegetables

These foods should be eaten in their raw, living state.
For better food combination, eat fruits alone or with leafy greens.

20% Beans, Nuts & Seeds
10% beans
10% nuts & seeds

These foods should be eaten in their raw, sprouted state.
Vegetarian protein and fat sources come from beans, nuts and seeds.

To assist in gleaning a clearer understanding of what this would look like, imagine looking at a plate of food you're about to eat for breakfast, lunch or dinner. Simply put, 80% of the foods you see on your plate would be fruits and/or vegetables, 10% would be sprouted beans, nuts or seeds and 10% would be avocado, nuts or oil. 100% of your daily fare would be eaten fresh and raw.

Sprouted Beans, Nuts & Seeds
Fruits
Vegetables
Leafy Greens

But always keep in mind that this plan is best varied from season to season. Again, unless you live in the Bahamas or southern California, if it's summertime, you'll eat more fruits than you would in the wintertime. If it's springtime, you'll focus more on spring green foods like watercress, dandelion and sprouts; after all, everything is turning green and sprouting in the spring. In the wintertime, you'll eat more fats than you would in the summertime because you're not eating as many fruits. So learn to shift and change with the changing of each season.

To show you how really simple it is, here's a sample week of menu ideas:

A Sample Week

Breakfast Always eat seasonal fruits in the morning. Choose from any fruit salad or superfood fruit smoothie in the recipe section or create your own. Feel free to add 1/2 cup cultured nuts or seeds (recipe on page 217) to any breakfast meal or smoothie. In the summer, when fruit is seasonally plentiful, I simply enjoy eating one type of fruit at a time, such as a big bowl of mangoes or a huge piece of watermelon. But if it's wintertime, enjoy a green "energy soup" with fatty avocadoes. Again, shift with the changing seasons.

- Enjoy a bowl of mangoes or papayas, grapes or some watermelon, whichever fruit is in season.

- Enjoy a bowl of "energy soup" made with a handful of baby greens, 1-2 cups of bean sprouts (alternating between mung, lentil and green pea), 1/2 of an avocado, 1 whole apple (peel, seeds and all), 2 tablespoons of sea vegetables, such as dulse or kelp and fermented coconut water as described on page 217.

- Supreme Superfood Fruit Smoothie—create a delicious smoothie with 2-3 different fruits such as a whole apple, banana and orange along with a 2-3 cups of water. Go ahead...blend the whole fruit, seeds and all. Add your favorite superfood such as goji berries or acai powder.

- Try a Berry Blend—blend 1/2 cup fresh organic raspberries, blueberries, strawberries and blackberries with 2-3 cups of water; add a frozen banana and a superfood powder or juice blend. Go ahead...be creative!

- Take yourself to the tropics with a Tropical Treat—blend 1/2 cup fresh organic pineapple, mango and papaya with lots of fresh young coconut water and coconut meat. Add a banana, 1/2 cup cultured almonds and 2 tablespoons rice bran complex.

- Have a Green Smoothie—blend 1 bunch of stemmed dinosaur kale with your choice of fresh organic fruit, such as mango, banana, pineapple and/or orange with 24 ounces water. Add a tablespoon of your favorite green powder blend.

- Start your day with one of my favorites—juice 2 apples, 1 unpeeled lemon, 1 2-inch piece of ginger, 2 ounces wheatgrass juice; then take it up a "hot notch" with 1/2 habanero pepper.

  Note Green-leafy vegetables such as kale can be mixed in fruit smoothies and still be a great, easy-to-digest food-combining combo.

Lunch Try a large leafy green salad with your favorite sprouted beans, nuts or seeds. Choose any Level One & Two salad in the recipe section you wish or again, create your own.

- Organic raw zucchini pasta tossed with olive oil, crushed garlic, salt to taste, freshly-chopped basil and lots of cherry tomatoes cut in half, all served on a bed of olive oil and garlic with tossed Arugula.

- Organic raw zucchini pasta tossed with lots of pesto served with a green leafy side salad.

- A bowl of your organic heirloom grains tossed with avocados and red onion slivers.

- A large Caesar salad with a side of sprouted organic beans.

- Dinner: The last meal of the day is a very light fare. Here are a few sample meals that can be found in the recipe section of this book.

- Raw tomato-basil soup served with a rainbow salad.

- Pineapple gazpacho soup served with a small, chopped veggie salad.

- Frieze-radicchio salad tossed in lemon juice and olive oil vinaigrette.

- Greek salad with cucumber-dill soup.

- Large "Berry Good" salad.
- Salsa sandwich and sprouted beans.
- Large "Butter Me Up" salad with red bell soup.

The "Go Green" *EcoDiet* Summary

The *Go Green EcoDiet* daily menu, while general in its application, can greatly assist you to create a strong foundation from which you can receive optimal *Go Green EcoDiet* alkalizing potential. The following is a more detailed check list of the most important things to keep in mind as you begin your *Go Green EcoDiet* journey:

✓ Drink 4-6 fluid ounces of ionized alkaline water every 30 minutes throughout the day, *the rainforest way.* Feel free to add the juice of one lemon for that extra alkaline boost and flavor; it also helps to dissolve mucus waste.

✓ Vary your foods with each changing season.

✓ Drink a *Supreme Superfood* Smoothie or Energy Soup every morning.

✓ Drink 1-quart of freshly-prepared vegetable juice every day.

✓ Eat 1/2 cup cultured nuts or seeds every day as they are predigested proteins.

✓ For better digestion and assimilation, take a slow 20 minute walk immediately after you eat.

✓ Follow the circadian rhythm for what and when to eat.

✓ Eat organically and/or biodynamically locally grown fruits and vegetables.

✓ Along with fruits and vegetables, eat a variety of grains, beans, nuts and seeds every day.

✓ Consume the right kind of salt, oil and sugar as outlined in Chapter 5.

✓ Always under-eat. If your last meal of the day is at 5pm, consider waiting until 10am the next day to have your first phytonutrient-rich Supreme Superfood Smoothie.

✓ Fast one day a week for a 24-hour period on nothing but ionized alkaline water. As an example, the last meal you eat before your chosen 24-hour fasting period should take place no later than 6:00pm. The next day, drink lots of ionized alkaline water until 6:00pm., then break your fast with a fruit meal only; one fruit at a time is always best.

✓ Weed the "garden of your mind" of every acid thought that arises. A heart of gold is cultivated when you give thanks for all things, even when going through the greatest of trials. Gratitude alkalizes your mind as well as your body. It opens the gateway to a purpose-filled life. It turns sadness into gladness, denial into acceptance, chaos into order and confusion into clarity. Gratitude helps us make sense of the past, which brings peace into the present moment and a healthy life into our tomorrows. When you focus your attention on seeing the good in every person and in every situation, a blessed life will be yours.

To Your Health!

Toni Toney

PART TWO

Kitchen, Cook & Recipes

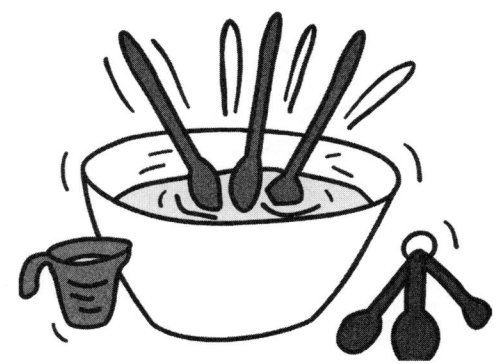

CHAPTER NINE

The EcoDiet Kitchen

Now that you've decided that the *Get Clean Go Green EcoDiet* lifestyle is for you, it's time to restock your kitchen with the necessary equipment, tools and foods. But before you do, you must first toss out the old before you bring in the new.

TOSS OUT THE OLD

Consider setting aside one full weekend to weed out any extraneous paraphernalia in your kitchen such as unmatched or chipped glasses, dishes, silverware, dull knives, warped plastic bowls and containers, or even those old scratched-up pots and pans that you just haven't wanted to part with. You may even want to include your partner or a friend or two in your EcoDiet kitchen renovation ritual. Clearing out the old to prepare for the new not only transforms your kitchen, in the end, it transforms you, too!

For greater efficiency, organize your countertop, cupboards and drawers. If your drawers are crammed full of items you haven't used in a decade, clean 'em out. Drawers that are difficult to open and close, and crammed full of useless stuff are time wasters. Or, if you have canisters full of white flour or sugar sitting on your countertop, open the lid and dump it out. Your body will never *Get Clean* if you don't clean your kitchen of all the acid-forming foods and products first. Be sure to also purchase *Go Green* earth-friendly kitchen soaps and cleaning products.

Now let's set up your EcoDiet kitchen with the specific tools and equipment you'll need for your new eco-logical way of eating.

TOOLS & EQUIPMENT

Like an artist who stands prepared to welcome the muse of creativity with his or her empty canvas, array of paints and specific brushes at his/her fingertips, you too, want to endow your kitchen with the essential tools you'll need for the delicious and alkalizing meals you'll be preparing. If your budget doesn't allow for a complete kitchen makeover all at once, start with the basics like a juicer and a high-powered blender that has enough RPMs to turn a hard nut into a creamy sauce or dressing, frozen fruit into sorbet, and cold vegetables into hot steaming soup. Then, when Christmas rolls around, ask "Santa" for the perfect food processor and a new set of culinary knives. Now let's take a look at each piece of equipment you'll want to purchase for your kitchen.

Juicer

Most health advocates would agree that the single most essential piece of equipment for a whole foods kitchen is a high-quality juicer. My two favorite juicers are the Breville 800JEXL Juice Fountain Elite 1000 Watts Juicer and the Green Star.

While most health advocates tout the Breville Juice Fountain as 'juicing made easy,' it is also highly acclaimed by Consumer Report. Over 50,000 Juice Fountain juicers have been sold worldwide. This Cadillac of juicers, with its patented extra wide feed chute, takes all the fuss out of creating wonderful fresh juice combos. No chopping or cutting needed; simply place the whole fruit, such as apples and carrots, down the feed chute. The Juice Fountain's powerful computer-controlled 13,000-RPM motor maintains the selected speed when juicing under heavy loads to give maximum juice extraction. The Juice Fountain's 2-speed electronic switch gives you greater control when juicing hard or soft produce. Simply switch to the low speed setting for fruits, which have a high water content such as watermelon, and the high speed setting for vegetables. And best of all, it's easy to clean, so I tout it as, "cleaning made easy!"

The Green Star is great for green leafy vegetables, sprouts, herbs and grasses such as wheatgrass. Its new and unique dual-stage juicing process achieves greater efficiency than most other single-auger juicers, which means that you get more juice from your produce. It works by filtering out juice during the initial crushing phase, before it can be reabsorbed into the pulp, and then squeezes the remaining pulp in the secondary pressing phase. This means that more juice goes in your cup and less stays behind in the pulp. Green Star's low-speed auger gently crushes and squeezes your produce so it will not heat up your juice and destroy life-giving nutrients and enzymes. With its included accessories, the Green Star also converts into a flat pasta or round noodle maker, making it a very versatile piece of equipment. It is durable, heavy duty, UL approved and will keep you equipped for juicing and raw food preparation for many years to come.

Blender

Most health advocates would also agree that the other most essential piece of equipment for a whole foods kitchen is a high-quality blender. My favorite is the Blendtec, also known as K-Tec. Most other blenders found in department stores just don't have the RPM power to turn hard nuts into a cream sauce or cold vegetables into a warm steamy soup. This high performance blender has the power to make whole food juice, sprouted nut butters, fruit smoothies, sorbets, ice cream and baby food, but it is best known for producing the best, most consistent results in taste and texture. The Blendtec has predesigned cycle settings. When a cycle button is pushed, it automatically speeds up and slows down, then shuts off when the cycle is complete. The Blendtec Total Blender has so much power (1500 Watts) it turns ice to snow and actually comes with an ice-crushing 8-year factory warranty.

Food Processor

Throughout the years, the food processor has become the most popular cooking appliance among gourmets everywhere. The Cuisinart PowerPrep is a professional grade food processor that outperforms any other food processor known. It dices, slices, chops, juliennes, minces, shreds, blends, purées...you name it; it does it. The name Cuisinart is synonymous with superior quality and innovation that gourmets have come to expect from their favorite kitchen tool. With the 14-cup PowerPrep Plus Food Processor, Cuisinart introduces a revolutionary new model. It boasts a new motor with an alternate speed for perfect dough mixing, a rounded housing for easier cleaning and handling, along with new safety features built into its bowl and cover. Not only will the Cuisinart PowerPrep save you a tremendous amount of time in food preparation, it will also enable you to prepare meals of uniform beauty. The Cuisinart PowerPrep comes in a heavy-duty stainless steel or white plastic casing. Whatever your individual preference, this piece of kitchen equipment is of immeasurable assistance in preparing the recipes included in this book and should be honored with a full time position on your kitchen countertop.

Mini Prep Processor

For small chopping, dicing, grinding, juicing or blending jobs you'll want a mini-prep food processor called the Magic Bullet. It is the perfect on-the-go piece of equipment, light, small and handy. It has a cross blade for chopping, grating and blending foods such as onions and frozen drinks, and a flat blade for whipping and grinding hard foods like beans, grains, seeds, nuts and spices. Both blades are made of stainless steel, so they are dishwasher safe and never need sharpening. This piece of equipment is inexpensive and a must for your *EcoDiet* kitchen.

Pots & Pans

Replace any of your scratched non-stick toxic cookware with natural non-stick and non-toxic cast iron; they may be hazardous to your health. These include cookware made from aluminum, Teflon, or copper. According to the Environmental Working Group, non-stick pans can contain PFCs, many of which breakdown into PFOA (Perfluorooctanic acid, also known as C8) in the environment and your body. Once in the body, PFOAs can circulate for years. PFOA is considered a carcinogen causing testicular, pancreatic, mammary, and liver tumors in rats. Evidence has shown that scratched non-stick pans, when heated, have the potential to kill birds because of the chemicals released. Plus, if the pan has even one scratch, you can ingest some of the toxic bits. Cuisinart has recently jumped onto the *Go Green* train with their new "Green Gourmet" Hard Anodized Eco-Friendly Nonstick Cookware. Featured at *Bed Bath & Beyond,* this new eco-friendly non-toxic cookware is both a great buy as well as a healthy choice. The ceramic-based coating makes it non-stick and scratch resistant. They are petroleum, PTFE (Teflon) and PFOA-free. While enameled cast iron cookware is also a great non-toxic alternative for healthy cooking, for most cooks, it tends to be heavy and hard to handle. It is still, however, a healthy choice.

Dehydrator

Food dehydration is a great way to create your own healthy and flavorful snacks such as dried fruits and vegetables or seed and grain crackers. It is also a great way to preserve the essence of a raw apple, as well as other fruits and vegetables because it doesn't subject foods to high temperatures associated with traditional food preservation methods like canning. Whenever a raw food is heated to an internal temperature of 118°F or higher, much of its nutritional value is lost, especially enzymes. Excalibur is the only dehydrator that has premium-quality features such as an adjustable thermostat, removable trays and door for easy loading, easy cleaning, pop-in, non-stick flex sheets, built-in on and off switch and drying performance that far exceeds all other models. While Excalibur makes a 5 or 9-tray model, the 9-tray is the one I most highly recommend, due to its vast range of dehydration.

Water Ionizer

While drinking lots of restructured alkaline water everyday makes a significant improvement in a person's overall health and wellbeing, the Kangen Water Ionizer, unlike most other ionizers on the market, also creates strong acid water (pH 2.5) that disinfects and sanitizes everything in your kitchen, from your countertop to your floor to chop blocks. This water kills HIV and other viruses on contact. Staph (MRSA), E. coli, salmonella and a host of other pathogens are destroyed in 30 seconds to a minute. Soaking foods such as berries, fish or chicken can be a great way to prevent any of these pathogens from entering your body. This ionizer also makes strong alkaline water (pH 11.5) that removes any pesticide residue from your produce while infusing them with negative ions that retard degeneration. The 11.5 water also emulsifies oil and grease in seconds, making clean up a breeze. I also use the 11.5 to make my salad dressings: with this supercharged ionized water, oil and water *do* mix!

Knives

One of the most essential kitchen tools is a great set of knives. Dull knives can make food preparation monotonous, dangerous and tiresome. Serrated knives are great for slicing tomatoes and bread while a heavy chef's knife is excellent for chopping or dicing. When shopping for professional quality knives, give the Miracle Blade knives from Japan your first dollars. They are light, affordable, razor sharp and never need sharpening. Compare a set of Miracle knives for around $60 to the heavier classic knives, such as Cutco, Henckel or Wusthoff, at ten times the cost. They come with a lifetime guarantee and are available at most large department stores or online. These knives will be a gift to yourself that you'll appreciate for years to come.

Spiralo Slicer & Spirooli

Designed and imported from Germany, these vertical turning slicers create streams of raw vegetable spaghetti in minutes using zucchini, squash and various other hard vegetables. The interchangeable blade system is fast, safe and easy to use and the sturdy suction legs hold securely to your kitchen counter. Just insert your vegetable and away you go. It's fast, easy and fun to use. The kids love it! But use caution; the blades are sharp. The Spiralo Slicer stands vertically while the Spirooli is horizontal. They are the same tool with a different structure. You choose!

Joyce Chen Spiraler

Within minutes you can turn almost any firm fruit or vegetable into thin angel hair-like strands or long flowing curly ribbons. With the spiral slicer, it's fun and simple to prepare a raw zucchini angel hair spaghetti dinner served with your favorite raw tomato sauce.

Mixing Bowls

Select a large assortment of mixing bowls from small to large, bamboo to glass. The bowls I recommend are French designed glass bowls made by Arc. They come with plastic lids making them excellent storage bowls for your leftovers as well as easy to use mixing bowls.

Cutting Boards

When shopping for cutting boards, bamboo products are amongst the best. Bamboo is a fabulous material to use because it's 16% harder than maple, making it perfect for a cutting surface or tableware. Even more importantly, bamboo holds the promise of a sustainable, cost-effective and ecologically responsible alternative to the widespread clear cutting of our world's precious timberland. Bamboo is actually a grass that grows to a harvestable height of 60 feet in about 3-5 years, growing as much as two feet per day. It has an extensive root system that continually sends up new shoots, which means it naturally replenishes itself. Bamboo boards can be purchased at most department or kitchen stores. You'll appreciate having several sizes on hand for smaller and larger jobs.

Salad Spinner

A sturdy salad spinner is a must for making fabulous salads. Simply wash your lettuce with cold purified water in the spinner bowl, then drain, rinse and spin. If there is leftover lettuce, simply place the lid on top of the bowl, seal and refrigerate. Lettuces will stay fresh and crisp up to three days. My favorite spinner is made by Zyliss from Switzerland and can be purchased at most kitchen supply stores. It's zippy, sturdy and easy to use.

Storage Jars

Air-sealed glass jars are useful for storing grains, beans, nuts, green superfood powders, seeds, salt, sugar, snacks, dried fruits, etc. Depending on the size of your family, you'll want to purchase between fifteen to twenty jars. For convenience and easy storage, I prefer the glass square ones with pull-off or screw tops. Snack foods, such as nuts and dried fruit, and for raw cane sugar, salt, etc., are best stored in the pull-off top jars sitting on your countertop for quick and easy access. Screw top jars are best for longer storage items such as beans and grains in the cupboard. If your budget is low, don't fret. These jars can even be found at most dollar stores. Note that common mason jars, or re-used product jars with lids work fine as well.

Sprouting Jars

Sprouting is fun and easy and there are two economical ways to grow sprouts. First, there is the glass jar version that can be purchased at most health food stores in various sizes. I like the half-gallon jars with strainer lids as the perfect-sized medium for growing sprouts: not too small, not too large. Wide mouth mason jars can also be used with a lid made of a piece of cheesecloth secured with a thick rubber band.

Kitchen Scissors

Sturdy kitchen scissors are handy to have at your fingertips for snipping herbs and cutting up dried fruit.

Small Essentials

To better assist you in preparing alkalizing meals, include in your kitchen small essentials: spatulas, measuring cups, a garlic press, a vegetable peeler, a hand-held citrus press, cheesecloth, glass storage bowls with lids, strainers, and tongs.

PANTRY & REFRIGERATOR

The day I walked into a health food store for the very first time, it was like I had just stepped off an airplane into a completely different country. Everything was so foreign to me. To help you, I have created a handy replacement list of foods.

For those of you who haven't made the all plant food vegetarian leap yet, notice that you simply toss out all of your commercially-raised meats and replace them with organically-raised meats. And remember, the meat portion of any meal should only be 20% or less and your veggie portion should be 80% or more.

Also, for those who live a fast-paced, convenience-necessary lifestyle, I have listed my favorite bottled organic salad dressings and staples such as canned organic beans and various other healthful prepared items. For those who love to prepare food and are graced with the time, I have created numerous healthy, freshly made dressings and sauces in the recipe section.

But for now, feel comfortable restocking your empty shelves with the following delicious, organic whole food products and condiments.

Toss Out	Replace With
Junk food snacks	Organic whole food snacks
White bread	Whole grain sprouted bread
White rice	Brown or jasmine organic rice
White sugar	Raw sugar or raw honey
White salt	Celtic Sea Salt®
Coffee and tea	Herbal and/or green teas
Canned or frozen vegetables	Organic fresh vegetables
Margarine	Organic Buttery Spread – *Earth Balance*
Commercially processed oils	Organic cold-pressed oils (dark bottles)
Boxed breakfast cereal	Whole oats or raw granola
Distilled vinegar	Organic raw apple cider
Mayonnaise	Grapeseed Oil Veganaise
Bottled salad dressings	Organic bottled dressings
Soy sauce	Nama Shoyu Unpasteurized Soy Sauce
Commercial herbs & spices	Organic herbs & spices
Roasted nuts & seeds	Organic raw nuts & seeds
Dried fruit w/sulfur	Organic dried fruit
Commercial kitchen soaps & cleaning products	*Go Green* earth-friendly soaps & cleaning products

SHOPPING LIST

Organic Cold-Pressed Oils

Hemp Oil

Grapeseed Oil

Extra Virgin Cold Pressed Olive Oil

Sesame Seed Oil

Pumpkin Seed Oil

Raw Coconut Oil

Flaxseed Oil

Organic Breads

Sprouted Wheat Tortillas

Sprouted Whole Grain Sandwich Bread

Whole Grain Sprouted Manna Breads

Organic Heirloom Packaged Grains

Forbidden Rice

Jasmine Rice

Bhutanese Red Rice

Short Grain Brown Rice

Wild Rice

Basmati Rice

Kamut

Oats

Millet

Amaranth

Quinoa

Organic Sprouted Whole Grain Pastas

Kamut Fusilli

Brown Rice Spaghetti

Kamut Fettuccine

Italian Buckwheat Pizzoccheri

Vegetable Spirals

Kamut Spaghetti

Vegetable Shells

Brown Rice Elbow

Organic Sprouting Seeds & Beans

Broccoli

Clover

Diakon Radish

Sunflower

Wheat Berries

Adzuki Beans

Lentils

Garbanzo Beans

Mung Beans

Organic Butter Substitute

Organic Buttery Spread

Organic Milk Substitutes

Rice Dream

Almond Milk

Hazelnut Milk

Hemp nut Milk

Coconut Milk

Organic Raw Sugar

Raw Honey

Yukon Syrup

Rapadura Raw Cane Sugar

Grade B Maple Syrup

Brown Rice Syrup

Cane Sugar

Molasses

Organic Sugar Substitutes

Stevia

Organic Zero

Organic Raw Chocolate Substitutes

Raw Carob

Teeccino Coffee Substitute

Vanilla Nut Herbal Coffee

Hazelnut Herbal Coffee

Mocha Herbal Coffee

Almond Amaretto Herbal Coffees

Organic Herbal Teas

Living Qi Organic Matcha Green Tea

Green Tea

White Tea

Chamomile

Red Cherry Tea

Yerba Mate'

White Rose

Hibiscus

Twig Tea

Peppermint

Organic Herbs & Spices

Basil

Oregano

Dill Weed

Rosemary

Sage

Tarragon

Marjoram

Thyme

Bay Leaves

Parsley

Cilantro

Cumin

Curry

Celery Seed

Turmeric

Cinnamon

Cayenne

Chili Powder

Paprika

Poppy Seeds

Nutmeg

Chili Peppers

Fennel Seeds

Salt

Celtic Sea Salt®

Organic Sea Vegetables

Hijiki	Dulse
Arame	Wakame
Kelp	Dulse Powder
Kombu	Kelp Powder
Nori	

Organic Raw Nuts & Seeds

Unpasteurized Almonds	Pecans
Cashews	Pumpkin Seeds
Walnuts	Sesame Seeds
Pine Nuts	Sunflower Seeds
Macadamia Nuts	Flaxseeds
Brazil Nuts	Hemp Seeds

Organic Dried and/or Canned Beans

Lima Beans	Black-Eyed Peas
Pinto Beans	Black Beans
White Beans	Great Northern Beans
Garbanzo Beans	Mung Beans
Kidney Beans	Lentils
Navy Beans	Cannellini Beans
Adzuki Beans	

Organic Fermented Foods

Sauerkraut	Kim-Chi
Vegi Delight	Chutneys

Organic Fermented Foods

Tempeh
Miso

Nama Shoyu Unpasteurized Soy Sauce

Organic Food Staples

Whole and Diced Canned Tomatoes
Roasted Garlic Pasta Sauce
Roasted Garlic Tomato Sauce
Raw Olives
Organic Coconut Milk
Grapeseed Oil Veganaise
Salad Dressings
Salad Dressings
Raw Apple Cider Vinegar
Balsamic Vinegar
Red Wine Vinegar
Ume plum vinegar
Tomato Ketchup

Organic Mustards
Vegetarian Worcestershire
Sweet & Sour Sauce
Vanilla, Brandy & Peppermint Flavors
Sun-dried Tomatoes
Capers
Artichoke Hearts
Nutritional Yeast
Dried Organic Fruit
Dried Raw Organic Coconut
Raw Carob Powder
Boxed Vegetable Broth

Organic Nut & Seed Butters

Raw Tahini
Raw Almond Butter

Raw Walnut Butter
Raw Pecan Butter

Organic Snacks

Dried Fruit

Trail Mix

Organic Crackers

Spelt Crackers
Kamut Crackers

Dehydrated Crackers

Organic Produce

Fruits In Season
Vegetables In Season
Spring Mix Greens
Arugula

Watercress
Romaine Hearts
Sprouts Of Every Kind

Organic Supreme Superfoods

Green Powder
Goji Berries
Acai Powder
Camu Camu Powder
Rice Bran Complex

Maca Root Powder
Bee Pollen
Royal Jelly
Active Manuka Honey 16+

Green Soaps & Cleaning Products

Laundry Detergent
Dishwasher Detergent
Hand Dish Soap

Floor Cleaner
All-Purpose Cleaner

WHOLE FOOD GLOSSARY

Brown Rice Syrup is a healthful and allergen-free alternative to other sweeteners. Substitute rice syrup in place of sugar, honey, corn syrup, maple syrup or molasses. Try it in muffins, cookies, fruits salads and smoothies. It's great in just about everything.

Organic Maple Syrup is a largely unrefined sweetener made from the sap of maple trees, maple syrup is a reddish-brown, viscous liquid with a sweet distinctive flavor. When it comes to purchasing maple syrup, the higher the grade, the better the quality. If you can find it, Grade C is the best; Grade B is second, then Grade A.

Really Raw Honey is a creamy white honey that has a mellow sweetness without any harsh bite and has a delicious creamy spread. Really raw honey is an alive, raw whole food packed with highly nutritious pollen, propolis, enzymes, trace amounts of royal jelly, and bits of honeycomb. This unfiltered, unrefined, unheated honey is utterly extraordinary.

Rapadura is a sugar cane from field to package is squeezed dried and ground and is the only whole, dried juice of sugar cane where the sugar stream is not separated from the molasses. When the whole natural juice of sugar cane is dried, it retains most of its essential nutrients, vitamins and minerals. It has a mild, caramel-like flavor superb for baking and sweetening any food or drink.

Sorghum is a syrup made from the juice of some varieties of the sorghum plant related to millet and similar in appearance to corn. The juice from the plant is extracted and cooked down into delicious thick syrup. The syrup contains vitamins and minerals and has a flavor and texture similar to that of molasses.

Stevia is a perennial plant native to Brazil traditionally used as a sweetener in beverages. It is 30 times sweeter than sugar, so two drops of Stevia extract can sweeten one cup. Stevia is a great for diabetics and a wonderful substitute for artificial sweeteners.

Celtic Sea Salt® is an authentic, unprocessed whole food salt made from one of the most pristine coastal regions of France. Since 1976, Celtic Sea Salt has been harvested by the *paludiers* (salt farmers) of Brittany using a farming method that preserves the purity and balance of ocean minerals. Celtic Sea Salt is doctor recommended, more nutritious than table salt, quality certified, and has exquisite taste. Use Celtic Sea Salt® for all your cooking and seasoning needs, to enrich the taste of your foods while adding vital nutrients to your diet.

Tempeh is an ancient Indonesian staple food made from fermented, cooked soybeans. Because it is fermented, it is the easiest of all soy products to digest and provides many essential vitamins. Can be used as an animal protein substitute.

Manna Bread is a moist cake-like bread containing no added sweeteners, oil, flour, salt, yeast, additives or preservatives. Manna Bread has all the fiber and germ of the original whole grain. After germinating the grain for a period of time, they crush and form it into loaves, then bake it at extremely low temperatures.

Miso is a traditional Japanese food produced by fermenting rice, barley and/or soybeans with salt and koji, a fungus used in Japanese cuisine that ferments soybeans to produce miso and soy sauce. This thick salty paste is easy to spread and is fabulous for flavoring soup bases. When purchasing miso, remember that the longer it's been fermented, the better.

Raw Olives are grown and processed on an exclusively organic farm so they have never been exposed to chemicals or pesticides.

Grapeseed Oil Veganaise is a mayonnaise made from Grapeseed oil, a by-product of wine production, that is a natural food known to increase the levels of HDL (the good cholesterol) and lower the LDL (the bad cholesterol). And, it tastes great!

Nama Shoyu Unpasteurized Soy Sauce is a fermented organic, unpasteurized soy sauce with a full-bodied flavor and an exquisitely delicate bouquet, plus healthful live enzymes and beneficial organisms like lactobacillus.

Nutritional Yeast is a nutritional supplement popular amongst the health conscious, this product, loaded with naturally occurring B-Complex vitamins, is a wonderful ingredient to add to recipes or as a condiment when looking for that cheesy-like taste, without the cheese.

Apple Cider Vinegar is a vinegar made from the finest raw organic, unfiltered apples possible and is full of zesty natural goodness.

Ume Plum Vinegar is a festive condiment rich in organic acids, this vinegar is a treasured by-product from traditional pickling of Umeboshi plums with sea salt and shiso (beefsteak) leaf. It's ruby red, tangy and very salty.

Raw Coconut Oil is a vegetable oil extracted from copra (the dried inner flesh of coconuts) with a wide range of applications. Coconut oil constitutes 7% of the total export income of the Philippines, the world's largest exporter of the product. Coconut oil is a fat consisting of about 90% saturated fat. Unrefined coconut oil melts at 20-77°F and smokes at 350°F, while refined coconut oil has a higher smoke point of 450°F. Coconut oil has a long shelf life compared to other oils, lasting up to two years due to its resilience to high temperatures.

Teeccino is an herbal coffee blend of herbs, nuts, fruits and grains that are roasted, ground and brewed just like coffee. Dark, rich, and full-bodied, Teeccino brings you all the satisfaction of a robust brew with no caffeine reaction. Teeccino tastes mildly sweet from dates and figs, but only has 15 calories per cup. This herbal blend comes in various delicious flavors. It is caffeine-free, non-processed, high in heart-healthy potassium, is highly alkaline, thus it helps reduce acidity and restore alkaline balance. It is also rich in inulin, a soluble fiber in chicory root that helps improve digestion and elimination plus increases the absorption of calcium and minerals.

Sea Vegetables are saturated with vitamins, minerals and protein, yet low in calories. You can usually find plastic bags of dehydrated sea vegetables in health food stores, or in the Asian foods section of larger supermarkets. After rehydrating, you can chop them up and add them to salads, soups, stews or stir-fry.

Goji Berries are a highly nutritious berry native to southeastern Europe and Asia. By weight, a daily serving has more vitamin C than oranges, more beta carotene than carrots and more iron than steak. Beta carotene is believed to fight heart disease and to also protect the skin from sun damage. Goji berries are also a good source of B vitamins and antioxidants, which protect our cells against harmful free radicals. They're also rich in polysaccharides, which aid the immune system, have 18 kinds of amino acids, and are a rich source of potassium.

Camu Camu is a highly nutritious red/purple cherry-like berry that comes from a small busy riverside tree from the Amazon Rainforest in Peru and Brazil. This fruit offers astringent, antioxidant, anti-inflammatory, anti-pain, anti-viral, emollient and nutritive properties and contains natural beta-carotene, calcium, iron, niacin, phosphorus, protein, riboflavin, thiamin and the amino acids valine, leucine and serine. This makes Camu-camu invaluable for metabolic processes, including the formation of white blood cells, maintaining a healthy immune system, and support for the brain, lymph glands, heart and lungs.

Raw Carob is the *only* healthy alternative to chocolate. Unlike raw cacao used to make chocolate, carob is free from the stimulants caffeine and theobromine. It is naturally sweet, so carob products will generally contain substantially less sugar than their chocolate counterparts. The great thing is that raw carob powder can be substituted for cocoa powder in any recipe.

Hemp Seeds contain all the essential amino acids and fatty acids necessary to maintain a healthy heart and mind. The seeds can be eaten raw, ground into a meal, used as a protein powder in smoothies, sprouted, sprinkled on top of salads, or made into hemp milk.

CHAPTER TEN

The EcoDiet Cook

In some cultures, *The Cook* receives the highest of honors. They are the king or queen of their station and are treated as royalty, and rightly so. The Cook is the one who prepares food for a meal, making it healthful and appetizing for all who sit at his or her table. To cook does not necessarily mean *to heat* food, as most believe. To cook actually means *to prepare*. Thus, The Cook is one who prepares food; the EcoDiet Cook is one who prepares food with eco-logical wisdom, which is the greatest gift we can give to ourselves as well as the ones we love and the ones we serve.

CONSCIOUS COOKING

Scientific studies conducted in 1930 by researchers at the Institute of Clinical Chemistry in Switzerland revealed that if food is cooked at too high a temperature, the body literally reacts to the food as a poison.

Premier Research Laboratories in Austin, Texas recently published these studies again, which clearly proves that after eating foods cooked at high temperatures, a rise in the number of leukocytes or white blood cells takes place. This rise in leukocytes demonstrates a strong immune response similar to a pathogenic infection. At first, this phenomenon, which was named *digestive leukocytosis*, was considered normal because everyone who was tested experienced the same results.

Researchers continued testing and found that eating unaltered, raw food, or food heated at low temperatures, did not cause an increase of the number of white blood cells. When testing many different types of foods, they found that if food was not overheated or refined, it caused absolutely no reaction. But if a food had been heated beyond a certain temperature (unique to each food), or if the food was processed or refined in any way, a rise in the number of white cells in the blood always took place.

Since it was not the eating of cooked food which caused digestive leukocytosis, but the eating of highly heated or refined foods which caused it, the researchers renamed this reaction pathological leukocytosis: *a reaction that is found only when the body is invaded by a dangerous pathogen or trauma.*

The study concluded that each food has a critical temperature. Above this temperature, the body no longer experiences the food as friendly. For example, the critical temperature for milk is 191°F. Today, milk and refrigerated juices are flash pasteurized or sterilized at 282°F, which is 100°F above the point at which the destruction of nutrients begins and where milk is no longer experienced as beneficial to the system but rather detrimental.

Highly heated foods, such as bread, crackers, chips, rolls, buns, muffins, cookies, cakes and bagels are typically heated at 350°F or higher. We can now understand why these foods create an adverse immune response. They are also nutritionally void, acid-forming and tend to congest the gastrointestinal tract, stagnate the elimination pathways and retard the lymphatic system. This is why people think they have allergies to various foods. Most food allergies are an immune response to this kind of perceived poison.

As we have previously stated, the worst offenders, heated or not, are processed foods: white flour, white salt, white rice and white sugar, and homogenized, pasteurized or preserved foods that were changed from their whole, natural form. The researchers discovered, however, that if these altered foods were thoroughly masticated or chewed, the harm to the blood could be lessened.

One Swiss study showed that the critical temperatures of several common foods range from 190-206°F. If a food is heated beyond its critical temperature, it produces pathogenic leukocytosis, an immune response to a toxic threat.

Food Critical Temperature

Water	191°F	Meat	194°F
Milk	191°F	Butter	196°F

Cereals	192°F	Oranges	197°F
Tomatoes	192°F	Potatoes	200°F
Cabbage	192°F	Carrots	206°F
Bananas	192°F	Strawberries	206°F
Pears	194°F	Figs	206°F

Pacific Research Laboratories reports, in response to this study, that if you eat foods that have been heated to temperatures at 190°F or less, your body will remain in a relatively non-reactive state. They found that highly heated baked foods such as bread could be replaced with low heated foods such as flat bread.

Flat breads are healthy, delicious and can be purchased at most health food stores under my favorite brand name *Ezekiel.*

For those who enjoy baked potatoes, try cooking them on low temperatures for longer periods of time. As an example, instead of baking your potato at 400°F in one hour or less, try baking it at 190°F for an extra hour or quartering your potato and cooking it in half the time. If you prefer steaming vegetables, simply keep your fire low which produces a lower temperature steam.

Obviously, your trusty kitchen thermometer and timer will serve to provide you with the feedback you need during your learning curve. Foods that have been cooked using low temperatures are not only more beneficial to your health, they are often more succulent and guaranteed to satisfy a gourmet palate.

THE HIERARCHY OF FOOD PREPARATION

Let's take a look at the hierarchy of food and how certain types of preparation can maintain or destroy their nutritional content. We will begin with the most nutritious way to prepare your food.

Raw, Living Organic Foods

Raw, living foods are foods that still have live enzymes. Organic raw, living foods rank first in their ability to supply your body with the highest quality nutrition available. These foods retain 100% of their nutrients. The organic raw, living food diet is the healthiest nutritional lifestyle you could choose. Raw, living foods can be juiced, sliced and diced, blended, sprouted, fermented or dehydrated.

Juicing

Freshly-prepared juice from raw fruits and vegetables retain 100% of their nutritional value. Healing centers across the world like Hippocrates Institute in Florida or the Gerson Institute in Mexico use juice therapy for healing and regenerating the sick. By separating the fiber from the rich concentration of alkalizing minerals, various nutrients and enzymes, this liquid food is like having a blood transfusion as it is absorbed into your bloodstream within minutes. It has been well established that freshly-prepared juice, because of its high concentration of minerals, enzymes and other essential nutrients, has the power to alkalize your system like nothing else. Many people who have followed juice therapy regimes have reported increased flexibility in arthritic joints, colds and flues disappear effortlessly, eyesight improves, and many serious illnesses often magically disappear! To receive maximum nutritional benefit, drink your freshly-prepared juice within 20 minutes of its preparation. Simply place your produce of choice in your juicer and within seconds, you'll be drinking your way to perfect health (pH)!

Slicing & Dicing

Sliced and diced foods retain 100% of their nutritional value. Due to a process called oxidation, however, it is always best to slice and dice your foods just before eating them. Once the skin of fruits or vegetables has been sliced open, oxygen combines with the enzymes and the nutritional content begins to decline through the breakdown of enzymes. Imagine for a moment what an apple looks like 20 minutes after you've peeled it. It turns brown because it has begun to decompose. This breaking down process is called oxidation. For this reason, raw foods are best consumed within 20 to 30 minutes of their preparation. While you may not be ready to eat a diet of just raw, living foods, they should be at least 50% of your daily diet. Simply slice, dice and eat!

Blending

Blended foods retain 100% of their nutritional value. The late and honorable Dr. Ann Wigmore, founder of the Hipprocrates Institute, used an array of blended foods, along with lots of vegetable juice and wheatgrass, for those with severe digestive problems. She estimated that over 90% of our population is unable to digest their food properly. Nutritionally rich, enzyme packed blended drinks will cleanse your body and supercharge your immune system, while giving your digestive system a much needed rest. Place the produce you desire to blend in a blender. Begin blending at low speed then gradually increase speed until you've reached your desired speed and consistency.

Sprouting

Sprouted foods retain 100% of their nutritional value. Easy to prepare, all you need is water, seeds, beans or grains and several large, 2-quart wide mouth glass jar containers with strainer lids or cheesecloth. Simply place 2-3 tablespoons of seeds, beans or grains in a jar. If you are unable to locate sprouting lids, cover the top of the jar with cheesecloth and secure it with a thick rubber band. Rinse the seeds several times in water then cover with lukewarm water; set the jar on its bottom and soak the seeds overnight. The next morning, drain the water; then rinse and drain again. Turn the jar on its side and place in a dark, draft free place. Keep the sprouts moist but not wet by rinsing them twice each day, morning and night. Swirl water around inside the jar of sprouts and drain. Depending on the variety of seed, the sprout or bud will appear in three to five days. It is during the first two to three days of germination that the nutritional value, as well as the alkalinity, of a sprout increases dramatically. It has been documented that by day three, the vitamin C content of soybeans increases drastically.

Fermenting

Natural lactic acid fermentation is one of the oldest and healthiest methods of food preservation. For centuries, the Japanese and Germans, in particular, have pickled their foods and kept them stored for over a year fermenting to maximize the development of enzymes and richness of flavor. Their wisdom also reflects the importance of the time needed to strengthen the colonies of friendly bacteria that we later consume to restore and maintain the internal integrity of our inner ecology.

Dehydrating

When foods are dehydrated, only 2-5% of their nutritional value is lost. With a dehydrator, not only can you dehydrate your own fruits and vegetables for delicious in-between meal snacks, but you can also prepare entrees as well as delicious whole grain crackers and tasty pizza crust. And best of all, it's simple. Before refrigerators and commercial preservatives, our ancestors practiced the art of dehydrating foods. They knew that by removing the water, the moisture content could be reduced to a level where unfriendly bacterial activity could not take place. Removing the water content allows for perishable fruits and vegetables to be stored for a long period of time.

Today, dehydrated foods have become very popular. Our fast-paced society is finding that dehydrated crackers, fruits and vegetables are ideal fast foods for in-between meal snacks as well as traveling and hiking. Of course, drying time will be different for each fruit or vegetable. Simply slice or dice your produce to desired thickness, place on the screen that comes with your dehydrator and turn the dial to desired temperature. In two days, you'll be enjoying the dried "fruits of your labor."

Freezing

When foods are frozen whole, sliced or diced even immediately after they are picked, the food loses anywhere from 5-30% of the plant's nutrient value, depending on how well the container they are stored in is sealed and how long the product has been frozen. If you are one of the fortunate few who have a backyard garden and you want to prolong your harvest by freezing, make sure to seal your food in airtight containers, preferably by using a quality brand vacuum sealer. Removing the air from the container is the key to nutritional retention and avoiding rancidity.

Steaming

If you're going to cook your food, steaming is by far the best possible method. Steaming can destroy anywhere from 10-60% of the nutrient value of the food, depending on the steaming temperature and the length of time, from low to high or 30 seconds to five minutes. Less is always better. Simply place your veggies in a steamer on low heat and steam. Just remember that as long as your food is moderately crunchy, it still has life. If it has gone limp, even though its been steamed, most of the plant's nutrients are most likely lost.

Grilling

Grilling is one of the tastiest ways to cook but can destroy from 10-60% of the food's nutrient value. Cooking outdoors with friends and neighbors can be fun as well as nourishing. However, skip the charcoal! Its smoke has been proven to be highly toxic and carcinogenic. Instead, use gas grills for all your grilling needs, both indoor and outdoor, or untreated wood chips from your local health food store.

Stir-frying

Stir-frying is a centuries-old Chinese style of cooking, usually employing a wok over high heat. Stir-frying is effective in retaining both the taste and most of the nutritional value of the food as it quickly sears the food at a high temperature for 1-2 minutes rather than cooking it longer on medium or low heat. One can throw just about anything into the wok and have it ready in a matter of minutes. Simply add a small amount of purified water and vegetable oil into your wok and heat. After the wok is hot, add desired vegetables and constantly stir for the entire cooking time. Stirring helps to keep the cooking temperature low and prevents the oil from breaking down.

Stovetop & Oven Cooking

Cooking can actually destroy anywhere from 40-100% of the nutritional value of food, depending again on the length of time and the temperature of the water.

Boiling food in hot water, for example, produces many undesirable changes. The main point to keep in mind is that *water too hot to touch is the real enemy of food value*. It removes water-soluble nutrients, breaks down enzymes and other nutrients into toxic compounds. These compounds bleach the color out of your food and rob it of its natural sweet flavor and nutrition. Stewing or baking your food at low temperatures in a small amount of water (or no water at all) actually increases the sweetness of food. Try it. Bake a beet, carrot, pineapple or banana in the oven at 200-250°F for several hours. The flavor goes off the chart. Or, put a lemon or lime in a moderate dry heat oven for a few minutes and notice that it becomes sweet like an orange. The low, dry heat intensifies the food's sugar content, but if you bake it too long, it becomes bitter.

Microwave Cooking

Microwave cooking destroys 90-99% of the nutritional value of your food. If you have one, recycle it. Microwave food is heated by a mechanical stimulation when microwaves bombard the molecules within the food, causing them to vibrate against each other causing friction. It's the heat from the mechanical vibration that cooks the food and in turn, destroys its nutritive value.

Leftovers

If there are leftovers at the end of a meal, make soup or throw them into the compost pile. Leftover foods are the perfect host for unfriendly bacteria, and the next lowest form of eating within the hierarchy of food preparation.

Processed Foods

Prepackaged processed foods are the lowest form of eating within the hierarchy of food preparation. Commercial food processing not only destroys 100% of the nutritional value of the food being processed, it further adulterates it by adding toxic preservatives and various other chemicals.

Summarizing the above information, another study published in the Journal of the Science of Food and Agriculture, revealed the results of four methods used for cooking broccoli: microwave cooking, boiling, high-pressure boiling and steaming. This is what they found:

- Microwave cooking zapped up to 97% of flavonoids (antioxidant compounds) that, when present, reduces the risk of lung cancer and heart disease.
- Conventional boiling killed 66% of flavonoids.
- High-pressure boiling nixed 47% of flavonoids.
- Steaming only caused a flavonoids loss of *less than 10%*.

While results will vary based on each food's chemical makeup, author Cristina Garcia-Viguera, professor of food science and technology at Campus Universitario de Espinardo in Murcia, Spain stated, "With steaming, the vegetable isn't in contact with water, so there's no direct leaching of antioxidants."

FOOD PREPARATION SUMMARY

Raw, juiced or blended foods

When fruits and vegetables are prepared raw, juiced or blended, virtually 100% of their nutrients remain intact.

Sprouted

When vegetables, beans or grains are sprouted, 100% of their nutrients are retained. Sprouted foods are easy to digest and are more alkaline and nutritious.

Fermented foods

When raw vegetables or grains are fermented, 100% of their nutrients are intact.

Dehydrated foods

When raw fruits, vegetables or grains are dehydrated, they only lose 2-5% of their nutritional value. If you purchase dehydrated fruits or vegetables, be sure they contain no added sugars or chemicals such as sulfur dioxide.

Frozen foods

When foods are frozen, they lose 5-30% of their nutritional value, depending on how they are packaged.

Steamed foods

When foods are steamed, they can lose 10-60% of their nutritional value. The value decreases according to steaming temperature and time.

Cooked or grilled foods

When foods are cooked or grilled, they lose 40-99% of their nutritional value, depending on how they were cooked.

Microwave

When foods are zapped with microwaves, 90-99% of their nutritional value is lost.

Leftovers

Cooked leftover foods are the perfect breeding ground for unfriendly bacteria, having no nutritional value.

Processed

When foods are commercially canned or processed, 100% of their nutritional value is lost.

CONSCIOUS RECYCLING

When it comes to an *EcoCook* in his or her *EcoKitchen*, one of the most important ingredients to remember to add to every recipe is recycling. Recycling saves our environment in so many ways. This is because much of the energy used in industrial process and in transportation involves the burning of fossil fuels like gasoline and coal, the most important sources of carbon and other greenhouse gas emissions into the environment. Additional benefits are derived from reduced emissions from incinerators and landfills and by slowing the harvest of trees, which are carbon sinks. In 2005, recycling reduced greenhouse gas emissions by 2.5 million metric tons of carbon equivalent (MMTCE) or 9 million tons of carbon dioxide.

In addition to greenhouse gases, recycling can reduce a range of pollutants from entering the air and water. By decreasing the need to extract and process new raw materials from the earth, recycling can eliminate the pollution associated with the initial stages of product development, such as material extraction, refining and processing. These activities pollute the air, land and water with toxic materials, i.e., ammonia, carbon monoxide, methane, and sulfur dioxides. Further reductions are achieved as a result of energy saving, thus reducing greenhouse gas emissions and other air pollutants. In addition to the greenhouse gas reductions mentioned previously, additional reductions of air emissions due to recycling total 587,000 tons. Reduced water emissions total nearly 9,000 tons.

The great news is that neighborhood-recycling programs have now made it convenient for most of us to recycle. Today, people are even being rewarded for recycling. Private and public programs are offering cash, gift cards and other rewards for eco-friendly behavior. So get on the "support the environment" bandwagon and start recycling today. Take advantage of these programs and encourage your neighbors, businesses and hotels to do the same. Step-by-step, we can team up and make our world a cleaner and healthier place to live.

CONSCIOUS COMPOSTING

Composting is a process that takes kitchen scraps and recycles them into a rich fertilizer for your garden and/or house plants. Food scraps and yard trimmings make up about 25 percent of the waste that U.S. households generate. Thus, composting your kitchen scraps greatly reduces the amount of waste that ends up in landfills or incinerators. And composting doesn't need to be complicated; after all, nature does it everyday. Simply create liquid compost…just by pureeing your food scraps in the BlendTec blender with enough water to make a thin soup-like mixture. Feed it to your plants. They, along with the environment, will be glad you did!

CHAPTER ELEVEN

The EcoDiet Recipes

The recipes in this section have been designed over the many years I owned my own gourmet vegetarian restaurant and taught hundreds of natural food preparation classes. While I have previously suggested a few of my favorite bottled organic salad dressings in the previous chapter to have on hand in your pantry, I have also included several easy-to-prepare, absolutely delicious salad dressings in this chapter that will increase your desire to eat more leafy-greens.

The key is to have two or three of your favorites on hand at all times in airtight Mason jars stored in your refrigerator, ready to whip out when you're in a fast-food hurry and need to quickly transform that ordinary plate of leafy greens into a 5-star gourmet salad.

The same holds true with sauces. You can almost always find a fresh supply of dairy-free pesto in my refrigerator. In the past, whenever I would come home from an all-day-outing tired and wanting to prepare something quick and easy, yet delicious, I simply cooked up (on very low heat) a medium-size serving of organic brown rice pasta, tossed it with pesto and served it up on a huge bed of Arugula greens and, *voila*, the perfect EcoDiet 80/20 Level One combo. But now that my taste buds desire a more 80/20 Level Two raw food fare, I simply put my Spirooli to work and make myself a large plate of raw zucchini noodles and toss.

So turn the page and begin this delectable *Get Clean Go Green EcoDiet* journey and alkalize your way to better health and a higher state of wellbeing.

Bon appétit!

Toni

LET'S GET JUICED!

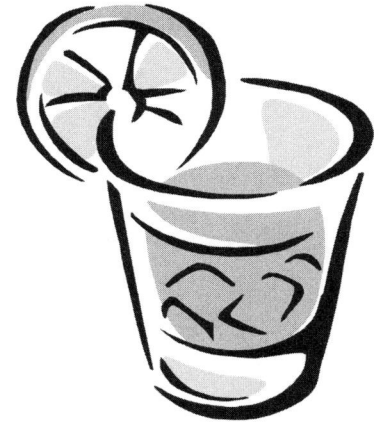

LEMON AID
Level One & Two

Did you know that Columbus took lemons on his long sea voyage to America because of their high Vitamin C content as well as other health-giving properties? That's why sailors were called limeys. Lemons have long been given to sailors to aid in the prevention of scurvy and are now enlisted in the prevention of cancer and rheumatism.

Grape Lemon Aid

1 quart green grapes
1 large lemon, unpeeled
Juice.

Apple Lemon Aid

6 apples, cored
1 large lemon, unpeeled
Juice.

Slushy Lemon Aid

2 lemons, juiced
1/4 cup raw honey
2 cups water
1 cup ice
Blend at high speed until smooth.

Warm or Cold Lemon Aid

1 cup lemon juice
4 tablespoons whole cane sugar
1 quart water
Blend at high speed until smooth.

Wheatgrass Lemon Aid

2 ounces wheatgrass
1 lemon, unpeeled
4 apples
2" piece of ginger
Juice.

ORANGE AID
Level One & Two

Juicy and sweet and renowned for its high concentration of vitamin C, it's no wonder that oranges have long been one of the most popular fruits in the world. Recently, some California chemists have even discovered that oranges are rich in a compound called citrus limonoids, which have been proven to help fight a number of varieties of cancer, including skin, lung, breast, stomach and colon.

Strawberry Orange Aid

5 Valencia oranges, juiced
1 pint strawberries, stemmed
Blend at high speed until smooth.

Avocado Orange Aid

5 Valencia oranges, juiced
1 avocado, sliced and pitted
Blend at high speed until smooth.

Mango Orange Aid

5 Valencia oranges, juiced
1 mango, peeled and pitted
Blend at high speed until smooth.

Kiwi Orange Aid

5 Valencia oranges, juiced
2 kiwi, peeled
Blend at high speed until smooth.

Papaya Orange Aid

5 Valencia oranges, juiced
1 papaya, seeded and peeled
Blend at high speed until smooth.

Pineapple Orange Aid

5 Valencia oranges, juiced
1/2 pineapple, peeled and cored
Blend at high speed until smooth.

APPLE AID
Level One & Two

No wonder Eve was tempted to eat this "forbidden fruit." An apple holds a magical power that will open your intuitive eyes and make you wise. So go ahead, drink. I can guarantee that when consumed daily, these elixirs will keep the doctor away.

Ginger Apple Aid

4 large apples, cored
2" piece of ginger
Juice.

Orange Apple Aid

2 apples, cored
2 carrots
3 oranges
Juice.

Waldorf Apple Aid

4 apples, cored
3 stalks celery
1 dash cinnamon
Juice.

Sweet Green Apple Aid

4 apples, cored
3 stalks celery
2 handfuls green grapes
Juice.

Raspberry Apple Aid

3 apples, juiced
6 ounces raspberries
Blend at high speed until smooth.

"ECOJUICE" RECIPES
Level One & Two

If you'll drink at least 1 quart of these freshly-prepared fruit and vegetable juices everyday for the next year and every year thereafter, nature will go to work and perform miracles. Bottoms up!

Grasshopper
2 ounces wheatgrass juice
2 Fiji apples
1 lemon, unpeeled
1" piece of ginger
Juice.

Raw Potassium Broth
1/2 bunch spinach
1/2 bunch parsley
3 stalks celery
6 carrots
Juice.

The Alkalizer
8 carrots
2 stalks celery
1/2 bunch parsley
1/2 bunch watercress
1/2 bunch spinach
Juice.

Liver Cleanser
2 apples
2 beets
7 celery stalks
6 carrots
1" piece of ginger
Juice.

Bile Flow
6 carrots
2 granny smith apples
Juice.

Intestinal Care
1 bunch spinach
8 carrots
Juice.

Liver/Gallbladder Cleanser
3 apples
2 beets
1 whole lemon
1" piece ginger
1 whole jalapeno pepper
Juice.

Sinus Socker
8 carrots
2 stalks celery
4 radishes
1 small piece horseradish
Juice.

Garden Greens
8 stalks celery
1/4 head leaf lettuce
1/2 bunch spinach
1/2 bunch parsley
Juice.

Insulin Regulator
8 carrots
1/2 head Romaine lettuce
1 pint string beans
5 Brussels sprouts
Juice.

Get It Up
1/2 bunch spinach
1/4 head leaf lettuce
Juice.

Eye See
8 carrots
3 stalks celery
1/4 head endive
1/2 bunch parsley
Juice.

Piles Upon Piles
8 carrots
1/2 bunch spinach
1/2 turnip
1 bunch watercress
Juice.

Oxy Green
8 stalks celery
4 kale leaves
1 bunch parsley
1/2 bunch spinach
Juice.

Heart to Heart

8 stalks celery
1/4 head leaf lettuce
1/2 bunch spinach
Juice.

"Triple A" Alkalizer

6 carrots
2 apples
2 stalks celery
1/2 bunch parsley
1/2 beet
1 green bell pepper
1 red bell pepper
8 tomatoes
3 stalks celery
Juice.

Hi Sugar

8 stalks celery
1 pint string beans
Juice.

V-8 Engine

8 tomatoes
3 stalks celery
1 green pepper
1 cucumber
1/2 red onion
5 radishes
2 cloves peeled garlic
1/2 bunch parsley
1 cucumber
1/2 red onion
Juice.

FRUIT SMOOTHIES
Level One & Two

There's nothing like a fruit smoothie or two on a hot summer's day. In fact, on those really hot days, with the exception of drinking lots of ionized alkaline water, that's all I'll have. It's like drinking dessert all day, and I really like that idea.

Banana Date

2 cups water
1/2 cup almonds, blanched
1 frozen banana
5 medjool dates, pitted
1 tablespoon vanilla extract
Blend at high speed until smooth.

Berry Berry Green

3 oranges, juiced
1 banana
1 cup frozen blueberries
1 cup frozen strawberries
1 cup raspberries
Blend at high speed until smooth.

Carob Mint

1 cup water
5 medjool dates, pitted
1 tablespoon raw carob powder
1 frozen banana
1/8 teaspoon peppermint
Blend at high speed until smooth.

Pineapple Coconut

1/2 pineapple, juiced
1/2 pineapple, diced
1 cup ice
1 cup coconut meat
1 frozen banana
Blend at high speed until smooth.

Red, White & Blue

1 cup strawberries
1 frozen banana
1 cup blueberries
1 cup almond milk
Blend at high speed until smooth.

Tropical Delight

1 large mango, diced
1 frozen banana
1 cup coconut milk
1 small papaya
Blend at high speed until smooth.

Banana Berry

3 oranges, juiced
1 cup frozen mixed berries
1 pear
1 banana
Blend at high speed until smooth.

Peachy Cream

1 quart frozen peaches
2 cups almond milk
1 tablespoon vanilla extract
3 tablespoons raw honey
Blend at high speed until smooth.

GREEN SMOOTHIES
Level One & Two

*Consider starting every day the Go Green way! In search of the perfect human diet, Victoria Boutenko compares in her book, **Green for Life**, the standard American diet with the diet of wild chimpanzees. Even though chimpanzees share an estimated 99.4% of genes with humans, it's obvious that their diet is dramatically different from ours—the chimp's diet consists of green leaves and fruits. She suggests drinking lots of green smoothies: a blend of 60% fruits such as apples, bananas and mangoes and 40% green leafy vegetables like spinach, kale and lettuce. Now I know it sounds a little radical, but try one. All you have to lose is those unwanted pounds on your hips!*

Apple Ginger Kale

4 apples, cored
1" chunk of ginger, peeled
5 kale leaves, stemmed
3 cups water
Blend at high speed until smooth.

Berry Green

3 oranges, juiced
1 frozen banana
1 pint blueberries
1 bunch dinosaur kale, stemmed
Blend at high speed until smooth.

Banana Apple Spinach

2 bananas
1 apple, cored
1 cup orange juice
1 bunch spinach leaves
2 cups ice (optional)
Blend at high speed until smooth.

Pineapple Coconut Watercress

1/2 pineapple, juiced
1/2 pineapple, diced
1 bunch watercress
1 cup fresh coconut juice
1 banana
Blend at high speed until smooth.

Pineapple Watercress

2 cups fresh pineapple
1 bunch watercress
Blend at high speed until smooth.

Acai Green

1 frozen banana
2 oranges, peeled
1/4 cup Acai Juice
2 tablespoons green powder
Blend at high speed until smooth.

Summer's Ginger Green

1 or 2 bananas
handfuls greens like spinach,
or sunflower greens
1" chunk of ginger, peeled
1 1/2 cups water
1/2 avocado, sliced and pitted
Blend at high speed until smooth.

Blueberry Green Protein

3 oranges, juiced
1 banana
1 pint frozen blueberries
1 handful dinosaur kale, stemmed
1 tablespoon hemp nut seeds
Blend at high speed until smooth.

Alpha & Omega Greens

2 whole apples
1 whole cucumber
3 celery sticks
2 handfuls spinach
4 kale leaves with stem
2 cups sunflower sprouts
2 tablespoons ground flax seeds
1 whole avocado, peeled
1-2 cups water
Blend at high speed until smooth.

Victoria's Favorite

6 leaves red leaf lettuce
1/4 bunch fresh basil
1/2 lime, juiced
1/2 red onion
2 celery sticks
1/4 avocado, sliced and pitted
2 cups water
Blend at high speed until smooth.

Nuts About Greens

3 cups water
1 bunch Swiss chard
1/4 teaspoon Stevia powder
1 tablespoon Maca Root powder
1 tablespoon hemp nut seeds
Blend at high speed until smooth.

Green & Clean

2 whole apples
1 whole cucumber
3 celery sticks
2 tablespoons ground flax seeds
1 handful clover sprouts
1 handful spinach
1 green chard leaf
1/2 head Romaine lettuce
1 avocado, peeled
1-2 cups water
Blend at high speed until smooth.

Green Apple Spice

2 whole apples
2 big handfuls spinach
2 celery sticks
1" piece ginger root
1 whole cucumber
1 whole lemon
1-2 cups water
Blend at high speed until smooth.

Johnnie Apple Seed

1 whole apple
1 avocado, peeled
1 head Romaine lettuce
2 celery sticks
1 whole cucumber
3 Swiss chard leaves
1-2 cups water
Blend at high speed until smooth.

SUPREME SUPERFOOD SMOOTHIES
Level One & Two

Imagine a superfood drink, not a drug, powerful enough to help you lower your total cholesterol, reduce your risk of heart disease and cancer, and, for an added bonus, put you in a better mood. And did I mention…without any harmful side effects? So, "bottoms up"…drink your way to wellness!

Carob Malt Smoothie

1 Thai coconut
1 small banana, frozen
1/4 cup pumpkin seeds
2 tablespoons raw carob powder
1 tablespoon maca root powder
2 tablespoons raw honey
1/4 teaspoon cinnamon
dash of cayenne pepper

Open coconut. Pour coconut water into blender; then spoon out all the meat and place it into the blender. Blend on high speed until smooth. Add the rest of the ingredients and blend at high speed until smooth.

"Bee" Always Young!

1 Thai coconut
1 banana, frozen
1 teaspoon Royal Jelly
1 tablespoon Bee Pollen
2 tablespoons Active Manuka Honey 16+
1 tablespoon maca root powder
1 teaspoon raw carob powder
1/2 teaspoon cinnamon powder

Open coconut. Pour coconut water into blender; then spoon out all the meat and place it into the blender. Blend on high speed until smooth. Add the rest of the ingredients and blend at high speed until smooth.

Berry, Berry Good!

2-3 cups orange juice
2 bananas, frozen
1/2 cup goji berries
1 cup blueberries
1 cup raspberries
2 tablespoons acai berry powder
1 tablespoon raw carob powder
1 teaspoon chlorella powder
1/2 teaspoon of cinnamon powder
1 tablespoon raw honey
1 teaspoon vanilla extract
dash of cayenne pepper

Place all of the ingredients into blender and blend at high speed until smooth.

Lou's Strawberry Heaven

2 Thai coconuts
2 bananas
1 quart strawberries
4-6 tablespoons vanilla rice bran complex
1 tablespoon maca root powder
1/2 cup cultured nuts

Open coconut. Pour coconut water into blender; then spoon out all the meat and place it into the blender. Blend on high speed until smooth. Add the rest of the ingredients and blend at high speed until smooth.

Maca Momma

2 Thai coconuts
1 pineapple
2 bananas, frozen
1/2 cup cultured nuts
1 tablespoons maca root
4 tablespoons vanilla rice bran complex

Open coconut. Pour coconut water into blender; then spoon out all the meat and place it into the blender. Blend on high speed until smooth. Add the rest of the ingredients and blend at high speed until smooth.

Seeds of Change

1 cup apple juice
1/2 banana
1/2 cup blueberries
1 tablespoon acai powder
2 tablespoons vanilla rice bran complex
1 tablespoon flaxseeds, ground
1 tablespoon chia seeds, ground

Place all of the ingredients into blender and blend at high speed until smooth.

NUT & SEED MILK & CREAM
Level One & Two

Instead of cow's milk, why not try nut or seed milk, milk made from raw nuts and seeds? Raw nuts and seeds are best soaked in water overnight before blending, increasing greater enzyme activity and digestibility. Enjoy nut milks on cereal or in a smoothie or even in your favorite soup recipe. When adding nut or seed milk to a soup recipe, just be sure to not include the vanilla extract and dates or raw honey.

Nut & Seed Milk & Cream

1 cup raw nuts or seeds, any kind

4 cups water

1 teaspoon vanilla extract

6 medjool dates or 1/4 cup raw honey

Milk

Combine all ingredients in blender and blend on high speed until smooth. Strain through a cheesecloth or fine mesh strainer. For a thicker creamy option, reduce the amount of water up to half or until you've reached your desired consistency.

Cream

You can also make thick nut creams using almonds or cashews without the vanilla extract or sweetener for soup recipes such as cream of broccoli. This recipe calls for 50% nuts and 50% water: 1 cup blanched almonds or cashews to 1 cup water. These milks and creams can be stored in a glass airtight container in your refrigerator for up to 4-5 days.

Coconut Milk

1 cup water
1 cup organic unsweetened coconut

In a blender, combine water and coconut and blend on high speed until smooth. Strain through cheesecloth or fine mesh strainer. Can be stored in a glass airtight container, like a Mason jar in your refrigerator up to 4-5 days.

Cultured Nuts & Seeds

1 cup nuts or seeds

Soak 1 cup of nuts or seeds for 24 hours in purified water, pouring off the water and rinsing several times. Pour soaked nuts or seeds into blender along with 1 cup water and blend until creamy smooth. Add 1/2 teaspoon powdered probiotics and stir. Pour into a 1 pint-size Mason jar, cover the top with a paper towel and let sit for 4 hours at room temperature. Seal and store in refrigerator until ready to use or up to 3 days.

Fermented Coconut Water

4 young Thai coconuts

Open coconuts. Pour coconut water into blender; then spoon out all the meat and place it into the blender. Blend on high speed until smooth. Add 1/2 teaspoon powdered probiotics and blend on low speed for a few seconds. Pour into 2 pint-size Mason jars, cover the jar with a paper towel and let sit for 4 hours at room temperature. Seal and store in refrigerator until ready to use or up to 3 days.

FRUIT SALADS

In-The-Raw

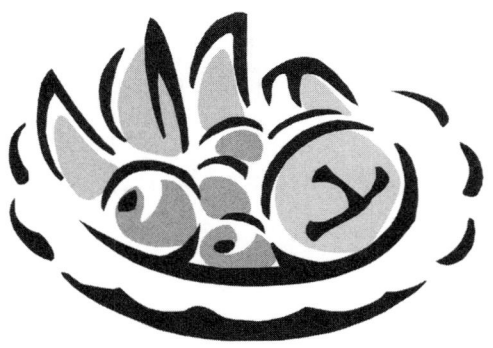

STRAWBERRY FIELD
Level One & Two

Spring

There's nothing like strolling through a field of strawberries that are brilliant red and ripe on the vine, lusciously calling to be eaten. The problem for me is that the temptation is always too great. I eat my breakfast in the field instead of my kitchen table. I make amends, however, by singing John Lennon's lyrics as I pick and eat...Strawberry Fields Forever.

1 pint strawberries, stemmed and cut in half
1 avocado, cut in half, pitted, cut into cubes and spooned out

In a small bowl, combine the strawberries and avocado, then toss with desired amount of Strawberry Sauce. Feel free to add a handful of your favorite green leafy lettuce.

Strawberry Sauce

1/2 cup strawberries, stemmed
1/2 cup water
2 tablespoons raw honey

In a blender, combine the strawberries, water and honey and blend on high speed until smooth.

PEACHY CREAM
Level One & Two

Summer

Peaches and Cream...what a sweet way to start the day. Peaches are a round stone summer fruit with orange or white flesh and fuzzy skin and come in three varieties: clingstone, with flesh that firmly adheres to the pit; semi-freestone; and freestone, with flesh that is easily separated from the pit. For those concerned about a more proper food combining fare, simply eliminate the almond cream sauce and replace it with one of your own favorite fruit sauces.

8 peaches, cut in half, pitted and sliced
3 bananas, peeled and sliced diagonally

In a medium-size bowl, combine peaches and bananas, then place into several parfait glasses. Pour desired amount of Almond Cream Sauce over the top and serve immediately.

Almond Cream Sauce

1/2 cup almonds, blanched
1/2 cup water
2 tablespoons raw honey
1 teaspoon vanilla

In a blender, combine the almonds, water, honey and vanilla and blend on high speed until smooth.

FIGS ON A MISSION
Level One & Two

Summer

The fig must have been the real forbidden fruit in the Garden of Eden. Its' tree-ripened flavor is way too tempting and completely off the pleasurable fruit chart. While the theory of the fig being the forbidden fruit in Eden can be disputed, it cannot be disputed that the first article of clothing worn by humankind was made of fig leaves. In fact, the fabulous fig has absolutely no origin, existing since the beginning of time. From Attica to Assyria and from Babylonia to Sumer, the fig has survived the fall of some of the greatest empires of the world. Commonly found in the peak of summer, figs are definitely on a mission.

1 quart fresh mission figs, stemmed and cut in half
1 banana, peeled and cut lengthwise into 6 pieces
5 dashes of nutmeg

On a medium-size serving plate, place the figs in a spoke-like circle with banana pieces flowered in the center. Remove one of the figs, cut it into small lengthwise pieces and place over the bananas. Pour desired amount of Fruit Sauce over the salad, then sprinkle the top with 5 dashes of nutmeg.

Fruit Sauce

1 orange, peeled
1 banana, peeled
1 kiwi, peeled
1 teaspoon raw honey

In a blender, combine the orange, banana, kiwi and honey and blend on low speed until smooth.

CRUISING THE CARIBBEAN
Level One & Two
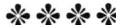
Summer

Tropical fruits are those that have their origin in the tropics and require a rather tropical or subtropical climate. In tropical areas where the temperature is relatively constant year-round, the fruits are still harvested seasonally. While there are hundreds of edible tropical fruits harvested in the summer, mangoes, papaya, pineapple and bananas are amongst my favorites. In fact, I ate them fresh off the tree in my backyard for breakfast every morning when I lived in Costa Rica.

2 large mangoes, cut lengthwise on both sides of pit, slice into 2-inch bite-size squares and spoon from skin
1 large papaya, cut in half, seeded, peeled and cut into 2-inch bite-size squares
1 small pineapple, peeled, cored and sliced
3 bananas, peeled and sliced diagonally
1/2 cup sunflower seeds, soaked overnight
1/2 cup almonds, soaked overnight

On three large dinner plates, arrange the mangoes, papaya, pineapple and bananas around the perimeter. In the center of each plate, place the soaked sunflower seeds and almonds, then drizzle blackstrap molasses and sorghum over fruit salad.

Sorghum Sauce
2 tablespoons blackstrap molasses
2 tablespoons sorghum

In a small mixing bowl, combine the molasses and sorghum and mix with fork

PINEAPPLE COCONUT BOAT
Level One & Two

Summer

Imagine cruising on a sailboat around the Hawaiian Islands. The sun is rising. You dock on a white sandy shore. You're hungry but come to realize you've landed on a deserted island. The landscape is lush; vegetation is everywhere. You see golden pineapples nested in a bush, calling out to you, asking to be eaten. Coconuts are everywhere, hanging on the vine and lying all over on the ground. Lucky you, you just happen to have a machete!

1 golden or white pineapple, cut in half
1 coconut, cut open with a machete or hatchet
2 bananas, cut diagonally
1/4 cup mint leaves, finely diced

On a cutting board, place pineapple with stalk still in place. With a long serrated knife, cut pineapple and stalk in half. Take a short serrated knife and hollow out the pineapple by cutting around the sides. Reach under the pineapple with your knife so that the flesh can be easily removed. When removed, put your pineapple boat to the side and with your short serrated knife, cut the pineapple into bite-size pieces. In a medium-size bowl, combine pineapple with banana, then toss; place fruit into your pineapple boat. Pour desired amount of Coconut Sauce over your fruit boat, then garnish the top with fresh mint leaves.

Coconut Sauce

Milk and meat of coconut
1 teaspoon organic vanilla extract
1 tablespoon raw honey

In a blender, combine the milk and meat of coconut, vanilla and honey and blend on high speed until smooth.

THE PERFECT MATCH
Level One & Two
❖ ❖ ❖ ❖
Summer

Who says greens and fruit and can't be eaten together? Chimpanzees eat them together in the wild all the time and our genes are almost identical to theirs. So go ahead...eat to your heart's content.

1 quart strawberries, cut lengthwise into thick slices
3 avocados, cut in half, pitted, cut into cubes and spooned out
1 head Bibb lettuce

In a medium-size bowl, combine strawberries and avocados. Separate lettuce leaves and place equally among 3 large wide-mouth serving bowls. Spoon fruit into the center of each lettuce leaf, then toss with desired amount of Orange Ginger Sauce.

Orange Ginger Sauce

2 Valencia oranges, juiced
1" chunk of fresh ginger
1 tablespoon flaxseed oil

In a blender, combine the oranges, ginger and flaxseed oil and blend on high speed until smooth.

PLUM GOOD!
Level One & Two

Summer

There's nothing like biting into a ripe plum. They are sweet, juicy and nutritionally packed. Just be sure to enjoy them while you can; most varieties are only available during the summer months.

3 plums, cut in half, pitted and sliced
2 cups red or green grapes, cut in half
1/2 pint strawberries, cut lengthwise into thick slices
2 peaches, cut in half, pitted and sliced
1 orange, peeled and sliced
2 kiwi, peeled and cut lengthwise into thick slices

In a large bowl, combine the plums, grapes, strawberries, peaches, orange and kiwi, then toss with the desired amount of Orange Liqueur Sauce. Place in a sealed airtight glass bowl and marinate for up to 6 hours in the refrigerator before serving.

Orange Liqueur Sauce

1/2 cup orange liqueur
1/2 cup orange juice
2 tablespoons raw honey

In a blender, combine the orange liqueur, orange juice and honey and blend on low speed until smooth.

FUJI & TAHINI ISLAND
Level One & Two

Autumn

The Japanese Fuji apple took America by storm in the 1980s. With the color, juice and firmness of a Red Delicious, this apple touts the flavor of an heirloom Ralls Janet. This apple is a late bloomer, often harvested in late September and October. For those concerned about proper food combining, simply eliminate the almonds and replace the Tahini Sauce with any sauce recipe your desire.

3 Fuji apples, peeled and cut into 1-inch chunks
2 kiwi, peeled and cut lengthwise into thick slices
3 oranges, peeled and cut into chunks
3 bananas, peeled and sliced diagonally
2 cups red grapes, cut in half and seeded
1/2 cup almonds, blanched (optional)

In a large bowl, combine apples, kiwi, oranges, bananas, grapes and almonds, then toss with desired amount of Tahini Sauce.

Tahini Sauce

1/3 cup Tahini
2 oranges, juiced
2 tablespoons sorghum molasses

In a small glass bowl, combine Tahini, orange juice and molasses, then mix with a fork until creamy smooth.

PEARS IN GREAT SHAPE
Level One & Two

Autumn – Winter

Ninety-five per cent of all pears grown in the U.S. come from Washington, Oregon and Northern California, where warm, dry summer days, cool nights, and wet winters combine to produce excellent fruit. Although pears are available at the supermarket year-round, they're at their peak of flavor in season. For summer pears, such as Bartlett, harvested in July and August, the season is brief. Winter pears, as presented in the recipe below, are available at the end of fall throughout the entire winter.

6 pears, 2 Bosc, 2 Lucas, 2 Vicar, cut in half, cored and cut into bite-size cubes

3 bananas, peeled and cut diagonally

1/2 cup walnuts pieces (optional)

6 medjool dates, cut in half, pitted and diced into small pieces

In a large bowl, combine the pears, bananas, dates and walnuts; pour desired amount of Carob Cream Sauce over the salad, then toss.

Carob Cream Sauce

1 cup almonds, blanched

1 cup water

2 tablespoons raw honey

1 teaspoon vanilla

2 tablespoons raw carob powder

In a blender, combine the almonds, water, honey, vanilla and carob powder and blend on high speed until smooth.

ORANGE 'U SPECIAL
Level One & Two

Autumn – Winter

Oranges originate from Southeast Asia, but are now available in warmer climates such as California and Florida, with the United States being the major producer of oranges in the world. Though I once believed oranges were named because of their color, the word orange actually came from the Sanskrit word naranga, which means fragrant. Depending on the variety, oranges are available all year long, with a peak season during the winter months.

3 oranges, peeled and cut into 1-inch cubes
2 avocados, cut in half, pitted, cut into cubes and spooned out
1/2 cup red onion, sliced in 1/2 slivers
1 package mixed salad greens

In a large bowl, combine the oranges, avocados, onion, and salad greens; pour desired amount of Orange Honey Sauce over the salad, then toss.

Orange Honey Sauce

1 orange, juiced
1/2 lime, juiced
1 tablespoon raw honey
1 cup cilantro leaves
1 garlic clove, peeled
1 small chunk of fresh ginger
1/2 cup olive oil

In a blender, combine orange, lime juice, honey, cilantro, garlic, ginger and olive oil and blend on high speed until smooth.

BETTER THAN WALDORF
Level One & Two

Autumn

Oscar Tschirky, the maître d'hôtel of the Waldorf-Astoria, created the first "Waldorf Salad" in New York City in 1893. The original recipe consisted only of diced red-skinned apples, celery and mayonnaise. Chopped walnuts were added later to this now American classic. Some prefer their Waldorf Salad made with yogurt instead of mayo, but I prefer it with honey lemon dressing.

4 Fuji apples, peeled and cut into small pieces
3 stalks celery, cut in half and finely dice top half, saving the bottom half for garnish
1 cup red grapes, cut in half and seeded
1 cup medjool dates, cut in half, pitted and cut into small pieces
1 cup raw walnut pieces

In a large bowl, combine apples, celery, grapes, dates and walnuts, then toss with desired amount of Honey Lemon Sauce. Divide equally into 3 tall serving bowls. Cut the remaining celery halfway down the stalk into 5 fan-like slices. Bottom half can be used for a spoon.

Honey Lemon Sauce

1 whole lemon, unpeeled
1/4 cup raw honey
1/4 cup water

In a blender, combine the lemon, honey and water and blend on high speed until smooth.

HONEY DEW YOU LOVE ME?
Level One & Two
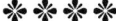
Autumn – Winter

In season, honeydews from California are the best, especially if the one you've just picked is ripe and ready to eat. To find that one and only special one, look for a golden color melon that has developed a bit of brown freckling on the rind. When you hold it in your hand, does it feel sticky? The stickiness indicates that it's loaded with sugar. Yummy...now let's have a ball!

3 melons, 1 honeydew, 1 cantaloupe and 1 canary melon, cut in half, seeded and
    scooped out into melon balls
Mint leaves for garnish
In a medium-size bowl, combine the melon balls; pour desired amount of Lime
Sauce, then toss and garnish with mint leaves.

Lime Sauce

1 lime, juiced
zest of one lime, green part only
1/4 cup raw honey

In a small bowl, whisk lime, honey and zest until creamy smooth.

LET'S GO ON A DATE, HONEY!
Level One & Two

Anytime

Honey dates are a soft, creamy-textured, sweet-tasting delight that literally melt in your mouth. And the good thing is, they are available throughout every season. So honey, let's go on a date, anytime, anywhere.

5 bananas, peeled and mashed

3 red apples, cut in half, cored and julienned

1 teaspoon cinnamon

In a medium-size bowl, place bananas; mash them with a wide-prong fork, leaving some bite-size chunks. Top with apples. Pour desired amount of Honey Date Sauce over the top, then sprinkle with cinnamon.

Honey Date Sauce

1 cup honey dates, cut in half and pitted

1 cup water

In a blender, combine the dates water and blend on high speed until smooth.

SALSAS & SANDWICHES

In-The-Raw

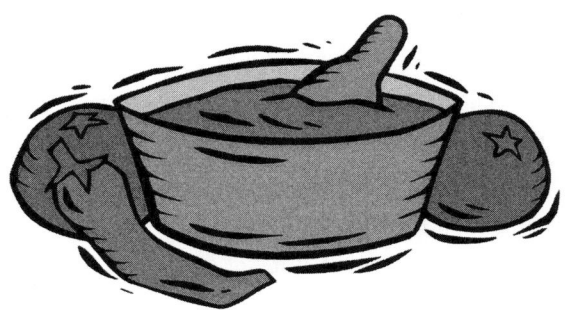

MANGO SALSA
Level One & Two
❖ ❖ ❖ ❖
Summer

This salsa can be served many ways: try it on a slice of roasted eggplant or, for a raw delight, simply spoon it into your favorite lettuce leaf. Before understanding the wisdom of healthy food combining, some of you may have even enjoyed fruit salsa with fish, beans and rice. But remember, if you combine fruit with protein your digestive system may not be too happy. I like my salsa best when it's served in a leafy green lettuce leaf.

2 ripe yet firm mangoes, cut lengthwise on both sides of pit, slice into 2-inch bite-
     size squares and spoon from skin
1 cup cucumber, peeled, seeded and finely diced
1 cup vine-ripe tomatoes, finely diced
1/3 cup red onion, finely chopped
3/4 cup red bell peppers, finely chopped
3 tablespoons cilantro leaves, minced
1 serrano chile, cut in half, seeded and minced
1/2 lime, juiced
Salt to taste
1 head leafy green lettuce, separate leaves (optional)

In a large bowl, combine the mango, cucumber, tomatoes, red onion, bell peppers, cilantro, serrano chile, lime juice and salt, then toss. Transfer to a sealed airtight bowl, seal and let sit several hours before serving to give all of the flavors time to merge into a fabulously tasteful delight. Serve wrapped inside your favorite leafy green lettuce leaf.

FIG FUJI SALSA
Level One & Two
❄ ❄ ❄ ❄
Summer

Figs are believed to have been originally cultivated in Egypt. They then spread to ancient Greece where they became a staple food within the Greek traditional diet.

2 Fuji apples, peeled, cut in half, cored and diced
1 cup fresh figs, cut in quarters
1/2 cup red onion, finely chopped
1 cup green bell pepper, finely chopped
1 tablespoon fresh ginger, grated
1 serrano chile, cut in half, seeded and finely chopped
1/2 cup roasted, spicy piñata pumpkin seeds
1 lime, juiced
1 head leafy green lettuce, separate leaves (optional)

In a large bowl, combine the apples, figs, onion, bell pepper, ginger, serrano chile, pumpkin seeds and lime juice, then toss. Transfer to a sealed airtight bowl, seal and let sit several hours before serving to give all of the flavors time to merge into a fabulously tasteful delight. Serve wrapped inside your favorite leafy green lettuce leaf.

CORN & AVOCADO SALSA
Level One & Two

Summer

What vegetable is more synonymous with the coming of summer than freshly picked corn on the cob? Corn has been a staple food in native civilizations since primitive times with some of the earliest traces of cornmeal dating back about 7,000 years. It definitely dates back as one of my all-time favorites. So if you're not eating corn in salsa, try it as a side dish, lightly sautéed in olive oil with green chilies and onions. You can even eat it raw.

3 ears corn, shucked, steamed, sautéed or raw and cut off cob

1 pint cherry tomatoes, sliced in quarters

1/2 red onion, finely chopped

1 jalapeño pepper, cut in half, seeded and minced

2 large avocados, halved, pitted, cut into cubes and spooned out

2 tablespoons cilantro leaves, minced

1/2 lime, juiced

Salt to taste

1 head leafy green lettuce, separate leaves (optional)

In a large bowl, combine the corn, tomatoes, onion, jalapeño pepper, avocados, cilantro, lime juice and salt, then toss. This recipe is delicious served with roasted eggplant and polenta, or simply served wrapped inside your favorite leafy green lettuce leaf.

TOMATO BASIL SALSA
Level One & Two
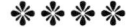
Summer

For a little Mexican salsa tradition, place a large scoop of your favorite guacamole recipe in the middle of a bowl and top it with this internationally renowned favorite.

2 vine-ripe tomatoes, chopped
1/4 cup red onion, finely chopped
1/2 cup red bell pepper, finely chopped
1/2 cup yellow bell pepper, finely chopped
1/4 cup fresh basil leaves, minced
1/4 habanera pepper, cut in half, seeded and minced
1/2 lime, juiced
Salt to taste
1 head leafy green lettuce, separate leaves (optional)

In a large bowl, combine tomatoes, onion, bell peppers, basil, habanera pepper and lime juice, then toss. Transfer to a sealed airtight bowl, seal and let sit several hours before serving to give all of the flavors time to merge into a fabulously tasteful delight.

Guacamole

3 large avocados, cut in half, pitted, cut into cubes and spooned out
1/2 teaspoon cumin
1/8 teaspoon cayenne pepper
1/4 cup cilantro leaves, chopped
1/2 lime, juiced
dash of salt

In a medium-size bowl, combine the avocados, cumin, cayenne pepper, cilantro, lime juice and salt, then toss to desired consistency. Serve wrapped inside your favorite leafy green lettuce leaf.

PINEAPPLE COCONUT MINT SALSA
Level One & Two
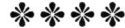
Summer

Try this Hawaiian style salsa on a simple leaf of your favorite alkalizing lettuce. Its flavor will open all of your senses for it is truly manna offered to us from the purifying fires of the volcanic gods!

1 golden pineapple, peeled and cut into 1/2-inch pieces
1/2 cup fresh coconut, shredded
1/2 cup red onion, finely diced
2 tablespoons orange juice, freshly squeezed
1 lime, juiced
1 serrano chile, cut in half, seeded and minced
3 tablespoons mint leaves, minced
1 head leafy green lettuce, separate leaves (optional)

In a large bowl, combine the pineapple, coconut, onion, orange juice, lime juice and serrano chile, then toss. Transfer to a sealed airtight bowl, seal and let sit several hours before serving to give all of the flavors time to merge into a fabulously tasteful delight. Serve wrapped inside your favorite leafy green lettuce leaf.

PERSIMMON SALSA
Level One & Two
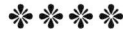
Autumn

Persimmons originated in China then spread throughout the Northeast Asian countries and then was later introduced to California and Southern Europe. Commercially there are two types of persimmons: hachiya and fuyu. They can be eaten fresh, dried, raw or cooked. Both evolve into their sweetest flavors when allowed to soften after harvest. They are one of my favorite autumn fruits!

4 ripe persimmons, peeled, cut into 1/2-inch cubes

2 tablespoons red onion, diced

1 tablespoon fresh basil, minced

1 serrano chile, cut in half, seeded and minced

2 teaspoons fresh mint leaves, minced

1 teaspoon fresh ginger, peeled and minced

1/2 lime, juiced

Salt to taste

1 head leafy green lettuce, separate leaves (optional)

In a large bowl, combine the persimmons, onion, basil, serrano chile, mint, ginger, lime juice and salt, then toss. Transfer to a sealed airtight bowl, seal and let sit several hours before serving to give all of the flavors time to merge into a fabulously tasteful delight. Serve wrapped inside your favorite leafy green lettuce leaf.

EGGPLANT SALSA
Level One & Two

Autumn

As a nightshade, the eggplant is closely related to the tomato and potato and is native to India and Sri Lanka. Because of eggplant's relationship with the nightshade family, it was once believed to be poisonous. While most people can eat eggplant without ill effect, for some, consuming eggplant as well as other edible nightshade plants (tomato, potato, capsicum peppers) can be harmful. Some sources state that nightshades, including eggplant, can cause or significantly worsen arthritis and should be avoided by those sensitive to them. But for those who aren't, enjoy!

3 medium eggplants, sliced lengthwise

1 large red bell pepper, cut in half and seeded

3 vine-ripe tomatoes, diced

1 clove garlic, peeled and pressed

1 red onion, diced

1 cup fresh cilantro leaves, minced

1 jalapeño, cut in half, seeded and minced

1/4 cup olive oil

1 lime, juiced

Salt to taste

1 head leafy green lettuce, separate leaves (optional)

Preheat oven to 200°F. Slice tops off of the eggplants and cut lengthwise into 1" slices. Coat sliced eggplant and red bell pepper halves with olive oil and salt. Place on a baking sheet and bake for about one hour, or until soft. Remove from the oven and place the eggplant and peppers into a sealed airtight glass bowl. Seal and let sit for 15 minutes to loosen the skin. Remove eggplant and peppers from the bowl, peel off the skins, dice and transfer to a large bowl. Add the tomatoes, garlic, cilantro, jalapeño pepper, lime juice and salt, then toss. Serve wrapped inside your favorite leafy green lettuce leaf.

SEASIDE SALSA
Level One & Two

Anytime

This recipe was designed for a macrobiotic salsa experience. Serve with lightly steamed kale and beans for an alkalizing appetizing delight.

1 package Arame Sea Vegetables, reconstituted

1 small carrot, julienned

2 cups red and yellow bell peppers, diced

2 cups yellow onions, diced

1 teaspoon ginger, finely grated

1 serrano pepper, cut in half, seeded and minced

2 tablespoons Nama Shoyu Unpasteurized Soy Sauce

2 tablespoons sesame seeds

1/2 teaspoon salt

1 teaspoon toasted sesame oil

2 tablespoons Ume plum vinegar

1 teaspoon raw honey (optional)

1 head leafy green lettuce, separate leaves (optional)

In a large bowl, rinse Arame in hot water, drain, then soak in hot water in a covered container for 30 minutes. On low heat, sauté carrots, bell peppers and onions for 3-4 minutes in a small amount of olive oil. Drain Arame after soaking. Add Arame to sautéed vegetables and cook over low heat for 2 more minutes. Add ginger, serrano pepper and soy sauce, then cook for 3-4 more minutes, or until excess liquid is gone. Remove from heat, then add sesame seeds, salt, sesame oil, vinegar and honey, then toss. Serve wrapped inside your favorite leafy green lettuce leaf.

FRUITS IN SEASON SALSA
Level One & Two
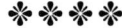
Anytime

With this simple recipe, you can make any type of fruity salsa you wish for any kind of season you're in.

1 cup strawberries, stemmed and medium diced

1 cup kiwi, peeled and medium diced

1 cup banana, peeled and medium diced

1 teaspoon fresh cilantro leaves, minced

1 serrano pepper, cut in half, seeded and minced

1 orange, juiced

1 lime, juiced

1 head leafy green lettuce, separate leaves (optional)

In a medium-size bowl, combine the strawberries, kiwi, banana, cilantro, serrano pepper, orange juice and lime juice, then toss. Transfer to a sealed airtight bowl and let sit several hours before serving to give all of the flavors time to merge into a fabulously tasteful delight. Serve wrapped inside your favorite leafy green lettuce leaf.

ALKALIZING APPETIZERS

Raw-&-Roasted

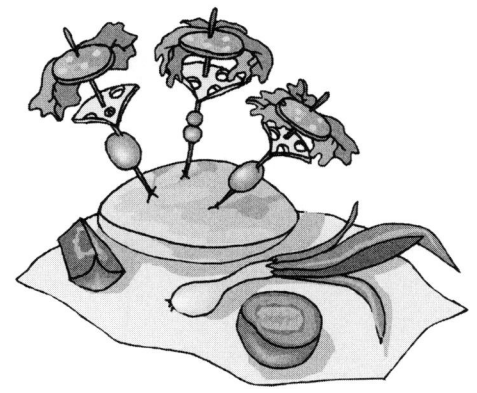

ASPARAGUS IN BELGIAN ENDIVE
Level One

Spring

Oh, the virtue of asparagus...one of nature's most perfect foods, springing forth in springtime, chock full of nutrients to revitalize us after a long winter's night. Bon Appétit!

24 small asparagus spears
2 heads Belgian endive
1 red bell pepper, cut in half, seeded and finely diced
Salt to taste

Snap off and discard tough asparagus ends. For culinary perfection, peel stalks with a vegetable peeler to remove scales. Leave spears whole and lightly steam in a steamer pan or serve raw. Separate endive leaves and place on a platter; place several asparagus spears in each endive leaf. Add finely diced peppers over the top for added color, then pour desired amount of Red Wine Vinaigrette over veggies and eat to your heart's content.

Red Wine Vinaigrette

1/2 cup red wine vinegar
1/2 cup olive oil
1 tablespoon tarragon

In a bowl, whisk the vinegar, olive oil and tarragon until smooth.

ARTICHOKES with CASHEW DILL SAUCE
Level One

Spring – Summer – Fall

Artichokes first appeared in southern Europe along the Mediterranean. The edible portion consists primarily at the base of the bud known as the heart; the mass of immature florets in the center of the bud is called the choke. Artichokes are extremely high in nutrients and are one of my all-time favorites. After removing them from the steamer, watch as their once hardened petals, now softened, opens up to you like a lotus to offer you its heart.

4 small artichokes

On a chop block, slice about 1" off the tip of the artichoke. Remove the smaller leaves toward the base around the stem. Cut excess stem, leaving around 1" on the artichoke. In a large pan, add approximately 2 inches of water and a bay leaf for added flavor. Insert a steaming, basket and place the artichokes bottom down. Cover and simmer at low heat for 30-40 minutes, or until the outer leaves can easily be pulled off. When ready to serve, dip artichokes in the Cashew Dill Sauce as a delectable appetizer or mini-meal.

Cashew Dill Sauce

1/2 cup raw cashews
1/2 cup water
2 tablespoons mellow miso
2 tablespoons lemon juice
1 tablespoon fresh or dried dill weed
1/4 teaspoon salt

In a blender, combine the cashews, water, miso, lemon juice, dill weed and salt and blend on high speed to a creamy consistency.

BROCCOLI with CASHEW TARRAGON SAUCE
Level One

Spring – Summer – Fall

Broccoli is a plant of the cabbage family and was an Italian vegetable long before it was eaten anywhere else. The Italians brought it to North America in the early 1800s but it did not become popular until the 1920s. Now, broccoli stands out as one of those vegetables that withstood the taste of time. Long touted as one of the healthiest vegetables one could eat, who would ever believe that broccoli could ever taste this good? The secret is in the sauce.

1 quart broccoli flowerets, steamed

In a steamer pan, lightly steam broccoli flowerets for 10 minutes, or until desired tenderness is reached. Transfer to a medium-size serving platter, then pour desired amount of Cashew Tarragon Sauce over the flowerets. Garnish with tarragon twig.

Cashew Tarragon Sauce

1/2 cup raw cashews
1/2 cup purified water
1 tablespoon mellow miso
1 tablespoon fresh or dried tarragon

In a blender, combine the cashews, water, miso and tarragon and blend on high speed until creamy smooth. For a thinner consistency, simply add more water.

BABA GANOUSH
Level One

Summer

This healthy, delicious Middle Eastern recipe can be used as a dip with pita bread or served as a side dish with tabouli and hummus. Sometimes I like to add a dash of "go green" parsley to this delectable dish. It gives it that special alkalizing touch.

1 eggplant, sliced into 2-inch rounds
1/4 cup raw Tahini
3 tablespoons sesame seeds
1 lemon, juiced
3 cloves garlic, peeled and minced
1 tablespoon vegetarian Worcestershire
1/4 cup olive oil
Salt to taste

Preheat oven to 200 degrees. Slice tops off the eggplant, brush with olive oil, pierce with a fork and place on a baking sheet. Cook for approximately 1 hour, turning occasionally until tender. Remove from oven, let cool and peel off skin. In a food processor, combine eggplant, Tahini, sesame seeds, lemon juice, garlic and Worcestershire, then purée. Transfer eggplant mixture into a medium-size glass bowl, add salt, then slowly stir in the olive oil.

TONI'S TABOULI
Level One

Summer

This delicious Middle Eastern recipe was inspired by a quaint sidewalk café I had the pleasure of eating at while touring the Hagia Sophia in Istanbul, Turkey. Not only is Tabouli one of Turkey's most famous traditional dishes, with hummus as a side dish, the two make a perfect couple. After returning home, I prepared it for my friends and served it as a wrap with green leafy lettuce leaves. It was a hit.

1/2 cup bulgur, soaked
3/4 cup hot water
1/2 cup parsley leaves, minced
1/4 cup mint leaves, minced
1/2 cup green onion, diced
1 large vine-ripe tomato, diced
1 cucumber, peeled, cut in half, seeded and diced
3 tablespoons olive oil
2 tablespoons lemon juice
Salt and pepper to taste

In a large bowl, pour hot water over the bulgur, cover and let stand for approximately 1 hour, or until tender and water is absorbed. When ready, drain excess water. Add parsley, mint, onion, tomato, cucumber, olive oil, lemon juice, salt and pepper, then toss.

HUMMUS with PARSLEY
Level One & Two

Anytime

Garbanzo beans and parsley...what a fabulous combination! Parsley originated in the Eastern Mediterranean region and, for more than 2,000 years, it has been known as a medicinal as well as a culinary herb. When combined with garbanzo beans, it immediately turns the acidifying beans into an alkalizing delight.

2 cups garbanzo beans, cooked, canned or sprouted (raw)

1/4 cup garbanzo bean liquid

1/2 cup parsley leaves, finely minced

3 tablespoons raw Tahini

3 garlic cloves, peeled

2 tablespoons Nama Shoyu Unpasteurized Soy Sauce

In a blender, combine the garbanzo beans (sprouted, cooked or canned) with a small amount of garbanzo bean liquid and blend on high speed until smooth. Add parsley, Tahini, garlic cloves and soy sauce, then blend again until creamy smooth.

BRUSCHETTA with ROASTED EGGPLANT
Level One

Summer

Bruschetta is a food whose origin dates to around the 15th Century from central Italy. When I took my very first bite of Bruschetta in Lake Como, Italy, I was raptured into flavor-heaven. The alchemy that opened up the taste of heaven's gate consisted of vine-ripened tomatoes and freshly chopped basil slathered on top a thick piece of grilled Italian bread rubbed with garlic and topped with olive oil. When I returned home, I hosted an Italian dinner party at my house. But because I'm a committed alkalizer, I replaced the acidifying bread with a more alkaline substitute...the eggplant.

1 eggplant, sliced into 2-inch rounds or 1 thick slice of grilled Italian bread

6 medium vine-ripe tomatoes, diced

4 cups fresh basil leaves, finely chopped

5 garlic cloves, peeled and pressed

1/4 cup olive oil

Salt to taste

Preheat oven to 200 degrees. Brush the sliced eggplant with olive oil and garlic. Grill eggplant over a low gas flame or bake for approximately 15 minutes on each side, or until tender and lightly brown on each side. While eggplant is cooking, in a medium-size bowl, combine tomatoes, basil, garlic, olive oil and salt, then toss. Remove eggplant from oven and top with tomato-basil mixture.

GRILLED PORTABELLA with APRICOT SAUCE
Level One

Anytime

Tonight, this meaty mushroom can be served like a grilled vegetarian steak with some added sweetness on the side. It's a gourmet appetizing treat for the highly discerning palate. This recipe was inspired by my favorite appetizer on the menu at The Inn of the Seventh Ray restaurant in Topanga Canyon, California. The great thing about this dish is that it's easy to make yet exquisitely gourmet.

6 portabella mushrooms, stemmed
1/4 cup olive oil
Salt to taste

Preheat oven to 200 degrees. Wash mushrooms with water, then rub with olive oil and salt. Place mushrooms in the oven top down on an open rack and roast for 30 minutes on each side, or until tender. Remove from oven and slice mushrooms into 2-inch slices. Serve with Apricot Sauce.

Apricot Sauce

1-12 ounce jar apricot fancy fruit spread
3 tablespoons brandy flavor
1/4 cup almonds, blanched
1/4 cup water

In a blender, combine apricot spread, brandy flavor, blanched almonds and water and blend on high speed until creamy smooth.

PORTABELLA PESTO PIZZA
Level One

Anytime

The largest of all the cultivated mushrooms known, portabella have open veils and flat caps that can measure up to 6" in diameter. Portabellas are actually mature crimini mushrooms with a meatier flavor, which is the result of a somewhat longer growing period. Fortunate for us, when the stem is removed, pesto can be served in its' tasty umbrella-style cap.

6 large portabella mushrooms, remove stems
1/4 cup olive oil
2 garlic cloves, peeled and pressed
3/4 cup basil pesto
1/4 cup sun-dried tomatoes
2 tablespoons pine nuts

Preheat oven to 200 degrees. Wash mushrooms with water, then rub with olive oil and pressed garlic. Place mushrooms in the oven on an open rack and roast for approximately 30 minutes on each side, or until tender. Remove from oven and top with pesto (see page 256) and sun-dried tomatoes. Bake for another 5-10 minutes, then remove from oven. Top with pine nuts.

GREEN BEANS with PESTO CREAM
Level One

Summer

For pesto lovers everywhere...this dish is for you. It'll rapture your sense of taste and lift your entire being into the heights of alkaline heaven!

2 pounds green beans, break off stems
1 tablespoon olive oil
3/4 cup basil pesto
1/2 cup pesto cream sauce
1/2 cup sun-dried tomatoes, chopped
1/4 cup pine nuts
2 tablespoons rice parmesan
Salt to taste

In a steamer pan, steam green beans for approximately 30 minutes on low heat, or until tender. Transfer to a large bowl, then toss with sun-dried tomatoes, olive oil and salt. Let sit for approximately one hour, then toss with pesto and Pesto Cream Sauce (see page 256). Sprinkle with rice parmesan, then mound in the center of a large white serving bowl and top with pine nuts.

BASIL PESTO
Level One & Two
❊ ❊ ❊ ❊
Anytime

Pesto is a sauce with its origin in northern Italy and has been a longtime traditional Italian favorite. Its name comes from pestâ, which means to pound or crush, the same Latin root as the English word pestle in reference to the sauce's crushed herbs and garlic. For those who have eaten at numerous American-Italian restaurants over the years, I'm certain you've found it on almost every menu. If you were to come to my home, you'll find that I always have a large mason jar topped to the brim with pesto. I love it on just about everything...pasta, grains, potatoes, veggies.

4 cups packed basil leaves, stemmed
1 1/2 cups olive oil
5 garlic cloves, peeled
1 cup pine nuts
1 teaspoon salt

In a blender, combine the olive oil, garlic and pine nuts; pulse on high speed for approximately 1 minute, or until the garlic and nuts are in small pieces. Be sure to not over-blend, as you want a semi-chunky consistency; not too smooth, not too chunky. Add basil leaves and continue to pulse, pulsing until the basil can only be seen as tiny flakes. Store in a sealed airtight glass container like a mason jar in your refrigerator until ready to use. For an added culinary delight, try topping your pesto off with a stream of Pesto Cream Sauce.

Pesto Cream Sauce

1/2 cup pine nuts
1/2 cup water
1 tablespoon pesto

In a blender, combine the pine nuts and water. Blend on high speed until smooth; add pesto, pulse and serve.

MANNA BREAD
Level One & Two
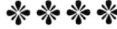
Anytime

Manna is the name of the only food eaten by the Israelites during their travels in the desert until they reached the land of Canaan. Manna is described as appearing each morning after the dew had gone while also appearing with the dew during the night, all of which implies nature's way of sprouting of the grain. Various passages only describe manna as being "good things" provided for us as sustenance. So if you're feeling adventurous and creative, you can make your own loaves of manna bread and have it on hand whenever you're feeling the pesto urge.

4 cups organic rye berries, sprouted

2 cups sunflower seeds, soaked

2 1/2 teaspoons ground caraway seeds

2 1/2 teaspoons ground dill seed

2 teaspoons salt

Soak organic rye berries in water in a sprouting jar for 8-12 hours. Rinse and sprout for 12-24 hours, rinsing every 2-3 hours. Soak sunflower seeds in a separate jar for 8-12 hours, then rinse. Place sprouted rye berries, sunflower seeds and spices in a food processor and blend for several minutes. Remove dough and form into 4-6 medium size 1" thick loaves and dehydrate for 12-16 hours. The bread will be moist on the inside and crusty on the outside.

PESTO PIZZA
Level One & Two

Anytime

When you've experienced pesto on sprouted Rye Manna Bread, you'll want to eat it anytime anywhere! Rye Manna Bread can be found at most health food stores in the freezer case. But if you feel ambitious, try making it yourself. It's easy, fun and delicious!

1-14 ounce loaf whole sprouted Rye Manna Bread
1 cup basil pesto
1/4 cup sun-dried tomatoes
1/4 cup pesto cream sauce

Knead bread and press flat into a 12-inch circle for a large raw pizza crust. Or, for individual pizzas divide the bread into 6 parts and make 6 smaller ones. Spread pesto (see page 256) on the pizza crust, drizzle a small amount of pesto cream sauce (see page 256) over the pesto and top with several pieces of sun-dried tomatoes.

RAW VEGGIE PIZZA
Level One & Two

Summer

For another raw foods manna bread pizza experience, be creative. Use your imagination. Try some finely chopped red, yellow and green bell peppers with red onions on your pizza. Delicious!!

1-14 ounce loaf whole sprouted Rye Manna Bread
1 pint Roma tomatoes, sliced lengthwise
2 tablespoons olive oil
1 teaspoon vegetarian Worcestershire
1 tablespoon organic hot sauce, or to taste
1 tablespoon Nama Shoyu Unpasteurized Soy Sauce
1 cup fresh basil leaves, chopped
1 cup raw kalamata olives, pitted
1/2 cup fresh chives, chopped into 1-inch pieces
1/2 cup sesame seeds
1/4 cup barley green
1/4 teaspoon salt

In a large bowl, combine tomatoes, olive oil, salt, Worcestershire, hot sauce, soy sauce and basil, then toss. Knead bread and press flat into a 12-inch circle for raw pizza crust. Spread sesame seeds and any kind of powdered green (such as barley green) on top of crust, then slather the tomato mixture equally onto the crust. Top off our pizza with olives and chives. It's "rawfully" good!

LINGUINI a la' RAW ZUCCHINI
Level One & Two

Anytime

This scrumptious dish is a great alkalizing alternative to pasta! It satisfies your craving for noodles without any acidifying effects. Try it. You'll not only like it, but I believe you'll love it.

4 firm zucchini, spiraled
1 cup basil pesto or marinara sauce
1/4 cup sun-dried tomatoes, diced

To make long noodles out of zucchini, simply use a vegetable spiral slicer like the Spiralo or Spirooli. To improve the texture of the noodles, try making them about six hours before serving, allowing them to sit in an uncovered bowl at room temperature. When noodles are ready, toss with pesto and sun-dried tomatoes or raw marinara sauce. Place it in your favorite bowl, then garnish with basil leaves.

Raw Marinara Sauce

3 vine-ripe tomatoes, blended
1 cup sun-dried tomatoes
1/4 cup onion, chopped
2 garlic cloves, peeled
1/4 cup olive oil
1 lemon, juiced
Salt to taste

In a blender, combine tomatoes, sun-dried tomatoes, onion, garlic, olive oil, lemon juice and salt and blend on high speed until smooth.

SALADS A LA' GO GREEN

Gourmet

Raw-&-Steamy

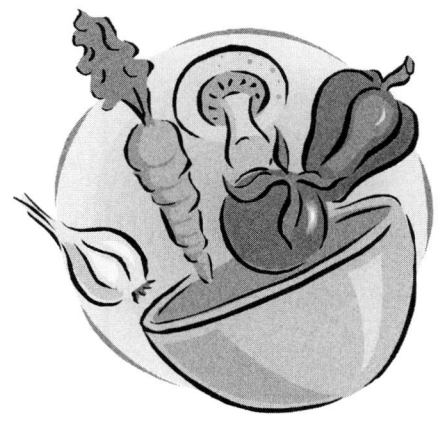

ITALIAN ARTICHOKE CAPER SALAD
Level One

Summer

The caper is a perennial spiny shrub that bears rounded, fleshy leaves and big white to pinkish-white flowers. A caper is also the pickled bud of this plant. The bush is native to the Mediterranean region, growing wild on walls or in rocky coastal areas throughout. The plant is best known for the edible bud and fruit, which are usually consumed pickled. Combined with the artichoke, this salad promises to be a perfect match!

1 small head frieze lettuce
4 Roma tomatoes, cut into quarters
1 cup large green raw olives
1 avocado, cut in half, pitted, cut into cubes and spooned out
1/3 cup organic capers
3 large radicchio leaves
6 artichoke hearts, cut into quarter-size pieces

In a large bowl, combine frieze lettuce with desired amount of the Vinaigrette Dressing; place into the center of a large serving platter. Toss tomatoes, olives, avocado, capers and artichoke hearts in desired amount of Vinaigrette Dressing. Spoon equal portion into radicchio leaves, then place in the center of frieze.

Vinaigrette Dressing

1/3 cup olive oil
1/4 cup balsamic vinegar
2 tablespoons tarragon leaves, chopped
Salt to taste

In a shaker bottle, combine olive oil, balsamic vinegar, tarragon and salt; shake vigorously until blended.

BRUSSELS SPROUTS & CAPER SALAD
Level One
✤ ✤ ✤ ✤
Summer

Brussels, Belgium, France or Rome...which country was the birthing place of the Brussels Sprouts, that leafy green bud that resembles miniature cabbages? Solve this puzzle and you're invited over to my house for dinner!

6 cups Brussels sprouts, cut in quarters
1 cup organic sun-dried tomatoes, diced
1/2 cup maple walnuts

Place Brussels Sprouts in a steamer pan and steam on low heat for approximately 10 minutes. In a large bowl, toss Brussels sprouts, sun-dried tomatoes and walnuts with desired amount of Organic Caper Dressing. Mound onto a salad platter.

Organic Caper Dressing

1/2 cup olive oil
3 tablespoons organic capers
2 garlic cloves, peeled
2 tablespoons red wine vinegar

In a blender, combine olive oil, capers, garlic and vinegar and blend on high speed until creamy smooth.

STEAMED VEGGIE SALAD
Level One

Anytime

Anytime, anywhere...this salad can be served as a main meal lunch or as a dinner party side. The Poppy Seed Dressing is what takes it to a gourmet 5-star experience.

2 medium carrots, peeled and cut diagonally
4 cups broccoli flowerets
4 cups cauliflower flowerets
1/2 pound mixed baby greens
1/2 pint cherry tomatoes, cut in half
1 cup clover sprouts
Salt to taste

In a steamer pan, steam carrots, broccoli and cauliflower for 10-15 minutes, then toss with salt. On a large serving platter, arrange baby greens, then top with steamed veggies and tomatoes. Drizzle desired amount of Poppy Seed Dressing over the top and garnish with sprouts.

Poppy Seed Dressing

1/2 cup raw honey
3 teaspoons ground mustard
2/3 cups apple cider vinegar
1/4 cup white onion, chopped
2 tablespoons poppy seeds
1 teaspoon salt
2 cups olive oil

In a blender, combine honey, mustard, vinegar, onion, poppy seeds and salt and blend on high speed until creamy smooth. Turn speed to the lowest setting and slowly add olive oil.

ROMAINE & ARTICHOKE HEART SALAD
Level One

Summer

Through the merging of these two hearts, romaine and artichoke, this summer salad can go down in your journal of salad memoirs as the best ever. The Thousand Island Dressing drizzled over every leafy bite takes this match to a new understanding of the "two becoming as one!"

2 romaine hearts, cut stem off and separate leaves

1 can organic artichoke hearts, cut into quarters

2 avocados, cut in half, pitted, cut into cubes and spooned out

2 vine-ripened tomatoes, diced

1/4 cup organic capers

1 handful broccoli sprouts

On a large serving platter, artistically arrange romaine leaves. Place artichoke hearts, avocadoes, tomatoes and capers in equal portions inside each leaf. Drizzle desired amount of Thousand Island Dressing over the top; garnish each leaf with broccoli sprouts.

Thousand Island Dressing

2 vine-ripened tomatoes

1/2 cup sun-dried tomatoes

1/2 cup pine nuts

4 tablespoons apple cider vinegar

2 garlic cloves, peeled

1/4 cup raw honey

Salt to taste

In a blender, combine tomatoes, sun-dried tomatoes, pine nuts, vinegar, garlic, honey and salt and blend on high speed until creamy smooth.

COSTA RICA POTATO SALAD
Level One

Anytime

In Costa Rica, huge avocados hang heavy from the bows of the trees. When I was there for 6 months, I would often pick one off a tree or buy one at the open-air market and have it for lunch or dinner. Avocados are like consuming "sweet cream d'la cure-all." Up until now, most Americans have feared the avocado's fat content, but the latest research shows that this Central American food is the food of choice for lowering cholesterol profiles. Nature made no mistake with this creation. So let me tempt you. Eat the fruit from the avocado tree. If you do, your eyes will truly be opened.

5 russet potatoes, cut into 2-inch bite-size cubes

1/2 cup celery, finely chopped

1/2 cup red onion, finely chopped

2 avocadoes, cut in half, pitted, cut into cubes and spooned out

1 cup cherry tomatoes, cut in half

1 tablespoon dill weed

1 teaspoon celery seed

1 small lemon, juiced

Salt to taste

1/2 head butternut lettuce, separate leaves

In a steamer pan, steam potatoes over low-heat for 10-15 minutes, or until soft. Transfer to a large serving platter and let cool to room temperature. In a medium-size bowl, combine the avocados, celery and onion and mash with a potato masher, leaving small chunks of avocado. Add the potatoes, tomatoes, dill weed, celery seed, salt and lemon juice, then toss until blended. Serve in lettuce leaves, topped with sprigs of dill weed.

BUTTER ME UP SALAD
Level One & Two
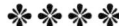
Summer

Butternut lettuce, what a delicate treat. Nature created these soft silky green leaves loosely packed around a small head, making it easy to turn each leaf into an alkalizing leafy burrito. And trust me, this tasty lettuce leaf salad is guaranteed to enchilada your tostado!

2 heads butternut lettuce

2 avocados, cut in half, pitted, cut into cubes and spooned out

1 jalapeño pepper, minced

2 cups cilantro leaves, stemmed and minced

2 cups yellow and red bell peppers, diced

2 cups ripe tomatoes, chopped

2–3 ears corn, shucked and cut off cob

In a medium-size bowl, combine avocado, jalapeño pepper and cilantro, then toss. On a large serving platter, artistically arrange lettuce leaves. Spoon avocado mixture in equal portions into each leaf. Top each leaf with equal amounts of bell peppers, corn and tomatoes. Drizzle each leaf with desired amounts of yogurt-mint dressing.

Yogurt-Mint Dressing

1 cup plain coconut yogurt

1/3 cup fresh mint, chopped

1 small lemon, juiced

1 tablespoon flaxseed oil

Salt to taste

In a medium-size bowl, combine yogurt, mint, lemon juice, flaxseed oil and salt. Whisk until blended.

BERRY GOOD SALAD
Level One & Two

Summer

Berries are the highlights of this summer salad. It's one of my favorites.

1/2 pound mixed salad greens
1 cup blueberries
1 cup raspberries
1 cup blackberries
1 cup strawberries
1/2 cup cherry tomatoes, cut in half
1 cup raw walnuts

In a large bowl, combine salad greens, berries, tomatoes and 3/4 cup walnuts, then toss with desired amount of Red Raspberry Dressing and stack in the middle of large serving platter.

Red Raspberry Dressing

1/3 cup raspberries (or raspberry jam)
1/3 cup water
1 tablespoon apple cider vinegar
1 tablespoon raw honey
1 clove garlic, peeled

In a blender, combine raspberries, water, vinegar, honey, and garlic and blend on high speed until well blended.

GREEK SALAD
Level One & Two

Summer

Greece is one of my favorite countries. I've spent a lot of time there, too. I actually spent 6 months on the island of Patmos last year and loved every minute of it. Served with thick slices of homemade sprouted bread to sop up the olive oil mixture at the bottom of your bowl, this Greek experience promises to be good to the last bite. So go ahead, try it without the feta cheese. You'll be glad you did!

2 large cucumbers, peel, cut in half lengthwise, scoop out seeds and cut into crescent
    moons

3 bell peppers, a combination of green and red, cut in halves, remove seeds and cut
    into 1/2 rounds

1 small red onion, cut into thin crescents

2 vine-ripe tomatoes, cut into quarters

1/3 cup raw Greek olives

1/2 cup fresh or dried dill weed

2 tablespoons fresh or dried Greek oregano

1/4 cup olive oil

Salt to taste

In a large bowl, combine cucumbers, bell peppers, onion, tomatoes, olives and herbs, then toss with olive oil and salt.

TOMATO STACK SALAD
Level One & Two

Summer

This heart-healthy tomato gourmet stack is a masterpiece. Layered with loads of olives, sprouts and pine nuts, it makes for an absolute evening epicurean affair.

2 beefsteak tomatoes, cut into 1/2" slices
1 cup pitted kalamata olives, chopped
1 pint sunflower sprouts
1/4 cup pine nuts

On a serving platter, we are going to create 2 tomato stacks, using 1 beefsteak tomato per stack, beginning with the largest slice first. In between each tomato, place olives, sprouts, and pine nuts, then drizzle with desired amount of Basil Vinaigrette. Repeat the procedure until you have 4 heart smart layers.

Basil Vinaigrette

1/2 cup olive oil
3/4 cup fresh basil leaves, stemmed and chopped
2 garlic cloves, peeled and pressed
1/4 teaspoon salt
1/2 teaspoon red wine vinegar

In a shaker bottle, combine olive oil, basil, garlic, salt and vinegar. Shake vigorously until well-blended.

OVER THE RAINBOW SALAD
Level One & Two
❋ ❋ ❋ ❋
Summer

This summer salad is colorfully satisfying and sends me "somewhere over the rainbow" on my list of salad expressions. The Miso Good Dressing gives it that final touch that literally takes it over the flavorful top!

1 head romaine lettuce, cut into bite-size pieces
2 beets, julienned
1 medium carrot, julienned
1 medium diakon radish, julienned
2 medium tomatoes, diced
1 green pepper, cut into small rounds and seeded
2 avocados, cut in half, pitted, cut into cubes and spooned out
1 package sunflower sprouts

In a large bowl, add lettuce, then arrange beets, carrots, diakon radish and tomatoes in mounds of four around the periphery of the leaves. In between each mound, place a handful of sunflower sprouts and avocados. Garnish with bell pepper rounds and serve with desired amount of Miso Good Dressing.

Miso Good Dressing

1/2 cup water
1 cup mellow miso
1 cup olive oil
1/4 cup apple cider vinegar
1/3 cup raw honey

In a blender, combine water, miso, olive oil, vinegar and honey and blend on high speed until smooth and creamy.

ALFREDO "Vegetablinguini" SALAD
Level One & Two

Summer

For a variety, this summer favorite can be served with marinara sauce, pesto, garlic pine nut cream or just plain olive oil, pressed garlic, salt, diced tomatoes, freshly chopped basil, and olives. Let your imagination take you wherever it will with this one.

3 yellow squash, cut in half, seeded and shaved
3 zucchini, cut in half, seeded and shaved
2 bell peppers, a combination of red and green, cut into halves, seeded and shaved
2 carrots, peeled and shaved
2 tablespoons olive oil
1/8 teaspoon salt

In a large bowl, shave squash, zucchini, bell peppers and carrots lengthwise into linguini-like strips with a potato peeler. Using a sharp paring knife, slice each strip into smaller 1/4" strips. Add 2 tablespoons olive oil and salt and massage for approximately 5 minutes, or until slightly wilted. Toss with desired amount of Alfredo Pine Nut Cream.

Pine Nut Cream

1/2 cup pine nuts
1/2 cup water
1/2 lemon, juiced
2 tablespoons olive oil
1 clove garlic, peeled
Salt to taste

In a blender, combine pine nuts, water, lemon juice, olive oil, garlic and salt and blend on high speed until creamy smooth.

WATERCRESS HIJIKI SALAD
Level One & Two

Summer

A love affair can be bittersweet, even with food. While watercress is considered a bitter leafy green, the Honey Mustard Dressing makes the bitterness disappear. My thought when creating this recipe was, "honey, you taste so-o-o-o good!"

2 bunches watercress, stems clipped

1/2 package Hijiki, reconstituted in hot water

2 tablespoons Nama Shoyu Unpasteurized Soy Sauce

1 small each red and yellow bell pepper, cut in halves, seeded and cut lengthwise
    into thin strips

1 medium diakon, julienned

1/2 cup maple walnuts

In a large bowl, soak Hijiki in hot water for 20 minutes. drain and rinse. Soak again in hot water for another 20 minutes; drain and rinse, then toss with soy sauce. Drain once again, return to bowl, then toss with watercress, bell peppers, diakon, nuts and desired amount of Honey Mustard Dressing.

Honey Mustard Dressing

1/4 cup organic stone ground mustard

1/4 cup really raw honey

1/4 cup raw apple cider vinegar

In a bowl, combine mustard, honey and vinegar and whisk until thoroughly blended.

BELGIAN ENDIVE SALAD
Level One & Two

Summer

Endive is deeply rooted in Belgian history. These tangy, tender and delicious white leafy greens were actually discovered there in 1830. Today, endive's fame and versatility has spread worldwide as more and more gourmet cooks and chefs turn to Belgium for the most flavorful, hardiest, tastiest gift to the world...Belgian Endive!

1 head red leaf lettuce, cut ends and separate leaves
8 heads Belgian endive, cut ends, cut in half and slice lengthwise
3 ripe pears, peeled and cut into thin slices
1 cup maple-glazed walnuts
Salt to taste

On a chop block, prepare red leaf lettuce and set aside; prepare endive. In a large bowl, toss endive, pears, and walnuts with desired amount of Maple Syrup Dressing, then transfer to a large serving platter. Artistically arrange red lettuce leaves, then mound Belgian endive mixture in the center of each leaf.

Maple Syrup Dressing

1/4 cup olive oil
1/4 cup red wine vinegar
1/4 cup maple syrup

In a shaker bottle, combine olive oil, vinegar and maple syrup. Shake vigorously until blended.

YIN YANG SALAD
Level One & Two
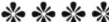
Anytime

The yin-yang balance of flavors explodes throughout your senses every time you take a bite of this salad, lifting you up and taking you far beyond this mortal existence. It's my favorite of all the salads served and inspired by Real Food Daily restaurant on Santa Monica Boulevard in Santa Monica, California. Stop by whenever you're in town. I know they'd love to serve you. Just be sure to tell them I sent you!

1/2 head Savoy cabbage, cut in half and finely shredded
1/4 head red cabbage, cut in quarters and finely shredded
1/2 carrot, julienned
1 1/2 cups cilantro, chopped

In a large bowl, combine cabbages, carrot and cilantro and toss with desired amount of Sweet and Sour Dressing.

Sweet & Sour Dressing

1/2 cup raw almond butter
1/2 cup water
1/4 cup olive oil
2 slices fresh ginger, peeled
1/2 cup brown rice syrup
1/4 cup brown rice vinegar
1 tablespoon Nama Shoyu Unpasteurized Soy Sauce
Cayenne pepper to taste

In a blender, combine almond butter, water, olive oil, ginger, brown rice syrup, brown rice vinegar, soy sauce and cayenne pepper and blend at high speed until creamy and smooth.

SPINACH & SUN-DRIED TOMATO SALAD
Level One & Two

Anytime

Add chopped sun-dried tomatoes to any recipe and it goes from a 7 to a 10 on the taste scale, especially this one. Then, if you pick your spinach from the field of a biodynamic farm like Whitted Bowers Fruit Farm in Cedar Grove, N.C., who grows their spinach from a biodynamic seed, you'll take this recipe leaps over the top of taste!

1 bunch spinach, stemmed

1/2 cup red onion, thinly sliced

1 cup organic sun-dried tomatoes, chopped

3/4 cup raw kalamata olives

1 cup clover sprouts

In a large bowl, combine spinach, onion, sun-dried tomatoes, and olives, then toss with desired amount of Poppy Seed Dressing. Transfer to a large serving platter and garnish the center with clover sprouts.

Poppy Seed Dressing

1/2 cup raw honey

3 teaspoons ground mustard

2/3 cups apple cider vinegar

1/4 cup white onion, chopped

2 tablespoons poppy seeds

1 teaspoon salt

2 cups olive oil

In a blender, combine honey, mustard, vinegar, onion, poppy seeds and salt and blend on high speed until creamy smooth. Turn speed to the lowest setting and slowly add olive oil.

CAESAR & CORNELIA SALAD
Level One & Two

Anytime

When Caesar married Cornelia in Rome'aine, his advisors told him that they were not the perfect match and was advised not to marry her. But Caesar was determined that she was his soul mate and refused their advice. He married her anyway. Because of their compatibility, they created alchemy and along with their committed love, they endured the taste of time.

1 head romaine lettuce, cut off end and slice
1 pint cherry tomatoes, cut in quarters
2 avocados, cut in half, pitted, cut into cubes and spooned out
2 large dehydrated raw crackers (optional)
Salt to taste

In a large bowl, combine lettuce, tomatoes, avocados, and crackers, then toss with desired amount of Cornelia's Dressing and salt.

Cornelia's Dressing

1 cup pine nuts
1 cup water
1/2 cup olive oil
1 lemon, juiced
3-4 garlic cloves, peeled
1 teaspoon salt

In a blender, combine pine nuts, water, olive oil, lemon juice, garlic and salt and blend at high speed until creamy smooth.

POPEYE & OLIVE OIL SALAD
Level One & Two

Anytime

Popeye built his strong muscular body on "biodynamic" greens alone. Smart guy that Popeye. Olive Oil thought so too!

1 pound fresh spinach, stemmed
1 granny smith apple, cored and cut into thin slices
1/2 cup red onions, cut into thin crescent slices
1/2 cup walnuts
2 tablespoons Rapadura sugar
Salt to taste

In a large bowl, combine the spinach, apples, red onions, walnuts, and sugar, then toss with desired amount of Olive Oil Vinaigrette.

Olive Oil Vinaigrette

1/3 cup olive oil
3 tablespoons red wine vinegar
Salt to taste

In a glass mixing bowl, combine olive oil, vinegar and salt, then whisk until blended.

NUTS for APPLE SPINACH SALAD
Level One & Two

Anytime

You've heard the cliché, "an apple a day keeps the doctor away," yes? Well, I bet whoever came up with that statement wouldn't be able to create one that could explain the benefits of eating apples and spinach together! One thing I do know for sure is that I'm nuts about this salad. In fact, this combo will not only keep the doctor away, it's so tasty you'll want to eat it everyday!

6 ounces baby spinach, stemmed
1/2 red onion, sliced thin
1 gala or Fuji apple, sliced thin or julienned
1/2 teaspoon salt
2 tablespoons olive oil
1/2 cup almonds, pulsed to a semi-coarse, powdery consistency
1/4 cup Miso Good Mayo

In a large bowl, combine the spinach, red onions, apples, salt and olive oil. In a blender, pulse almonds on high speed until a semi-coarse, yet powdery consistency is reached. Add to salad, then toss with desired amount of Miso Good Mayo Dressing.

Miso Good Mayo Dressing

1/2 cup Sweet White Miso
1/2 cup olive oil
2 tablespoons Nama Shoyu Soy Sauce
2 tablespoons apple cider vinegar
1/4 cup water

In a blender, combine miso, olive oil, soy sauce, vinegar and water and blend on high speed until creamy smooth.

SPIRALED SWEET POTATO SALAD
Level One & Two
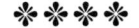
Autumn – Winter

One potato, two potatoes, three potatoes, four...five potatoes, six potatoes, seven potatoes and, believe me, you'll want more. This recipe is a sweet, spiraling gourmet salad delight.

7 sweet potatoes, peeled and spiraled
1 cup currants
1 cup raw walnuts
1 teaspoon cinnamon
1 pinch salt

Using the flat blade of the Joyce Chen Spiraler, spiral peeled sweet potatoes into long ribbons. Transfer to a large serving platter; add currants, walnuts, cinnamon and salt, then toss with desired amount of Halvah Dressing. Arrange salad into a tall luscious mound in the center of serving platter. Garnish with edible flowers.

Halvah Dressing

1/4 cup raw Tahini
1/4 cup raw honey
1 orange, juiced

In a small bowl, combine Tahini, honey and orange juice. Stir with a wide-pronged fork until creamy smooth.

WATERCRESS SPROUT SALAD
Level One & Two

Autumn

Every main morsel of this salad is birthed out of water. Watercress, native from Europe to central Asia, is one of the oldest known leafy greens. Thriving best in water, this rich alkaline leafy green is noted for its peppery, tangy flavor. Best of all, by weight, watercress has more calcium than milk and more vitamin C than an orange.

1 large bunch watercress, stemmed
2 large radicchio leaves
1 cup sun-dried olives
1 cup cherry tomatoes, sliced into quarters
1 cup organic artichoke hearts, cut into quarters
1 cup lentils, sprouted
Salt to taste
1 handful sunflower or pea sprouts

In a large bowl, toss watercress with Olive Oil Vinaigrette, then place in the center of a large serving plate. Set two radicchio leaves on top. Combine olives, tomatoes, artichoke hearts, sprouted lentils and salt in bowl, then toss with desired amount of Olive Oil Vinaigrette. Fill each radicchio leaf with salad. Artistically arrange sunflower or pea sprouts around the outer edge of serving plate.

Papaya Vinaigrette

1 cup fresh papaya
1/3 cup olive oil
3 tablespoons red wine vinegar
2 garlic cloves, peeled and pressed
    dash of water
Salt to taste

In a small bowl, combine olive oil, vinegar, garlic and salt, then whisk until blended. Use a dash of water, if needed.

WATERCRESS AVOCADO SALAD
Level One & Two

Autumn

Simply gourmet, this delectable salad is guaranteed to be the hit of any of your finest dinner parties.

1 bunch watercress, stemmed
1 avocado, cut in half, pitted, cut into cubes and spooned out

In a medium-size bowl, combine watercress and avocado, then toss with desired amount of Sweet Apple Dressing.

Sweet Apple Dressing

1/4 cup brown rice vinegar
1 tablespoon sweet onion, grated
1/4 cup Gala apple, peeled and finely grated
2 tablespoons Nama Shoyu Unpasteurized Soy Sauce
1 teaspoon raw honey
3 tablespoons sunflower oil
Salt to taste

In a shaker jar, combine vinegar, onion, apple, soy sauce, raw honey, sunflower oil and salt. Shake vigorously until blended.

GOLDEN ITALIAN SALAD
Level One

Summer – Autumn

The first moment I put a Yukon gold potato in my mouth, I knew I had just struck gold. Their golden, buttery-tasting flavor, coupled with lots of olive oil, garlic and salt takes this recipe straight to the top of any gourmet 5-star experience.

6 medium Yukon gold potatoes, cut in half lengthwise then into 1-inch wedges
4 red bell peppers, cut into halves, seeded and sliced into 1/4-inch strips
3 tablespoons olive oil
3 large garlic cloves, peeled and pressed
15 large garlic cloves, peeled
Salt to taste
4 cups loosely packed baby Arugula
Dash of olive oil

Preheat oven to 250 degrees. In a large bowl, combine the potatoes and bell peppers, then rub with olive oil and pressed garlic. Add whole garlic cloves, then toss. Transfer to a large baking pan, then bake for approximately 1 hour, or until potatoes are golden brown. Remove from oven. Transfer to a large serving platter, then salt to taste and let cool. When ready to serve, toss potatoes and peppers with Arugula, along with a dash of olive oil.

SOUP IT UP

Raw-&-Steamy

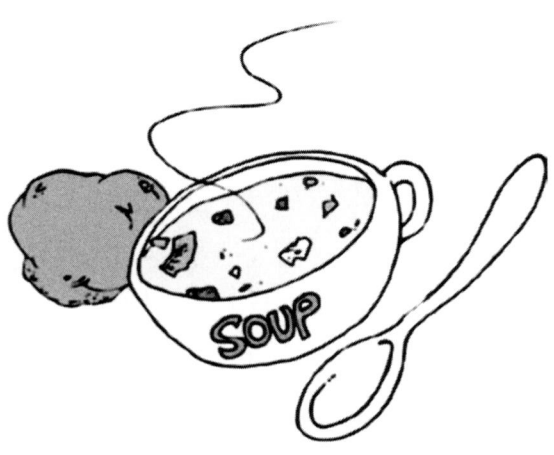

ASPARAGUS MISO SOUP
Level One
❖ ❖ ❖ ❖
Spring

In the first century, Pliny the Elder, an ancient author, naturalist and philosopher wrote, "asparagus, of all the plants of the garden, receives the most praiseworthy care." Its botanical species name, "officinalis" indicates its recognition as an official therapeutic herb. The herb has been highly valued and prescribed to cleanse, revitalize and strengthen kidney and bladder function. Some even say, "4 tablespoons a day will keep cancer away!"

1 bunch spring onions, diced

3 carrots, peeled, cut in half and sliced diagonally

2 tablespoons olive oil

1 pound asparagus, cut into 2" pieces

1 quart water

6 ounces sweet white miso

In a medium-size soup pot, add olive oil and sauté the spring onions and carrots on low heat for 10 minutes, or until carrots are tender. In a steamer pan, steam the asparagus for 5-10 minutes, or until tender. Transfer the asparagus to the soup pot, then stir. In a blender, combine water and miso and blend on low speed for one minute or until thoroughly blended. Pour miso-water into soup pot and stir. Cover and cook on low heat for approximately 10 minutes. Remove from heat and let sit for 30 minutes before serving.

HOT TOMATO BASIL SOUP

Level One

✤✤✤✤

Summer

There's nothing like a bowl of Italian tomato basil soup. Hot or cold, this soup is as easy as a summer breeze and just as delicious. Some believe that the secret to the richness of this soup is to use real butter and heavy cream. But I found another more alkalizing way...almond cream!

1 large yellow onion, sliced
2 tablespoons olive oil
5 vine-ripe pear-shaped Italian tomatoes, chopped
1 cup fresh basil leaves, stemmed and chopped
1 tablespoon red wine vinegar
1 cup organic vegetable broth
1 tablespoon salt
1/8 teaspoon black pepper

In a medium-size soup pot, add olive oil and sauté onion for 10 minutes, or until onion is translucent. Stir in tomatoes, basil and vinegar. Cover and cook for 10-15 minutes. Transfer to blender; add vegetable broth, salt, pepper and almond cream, then blend on high speed until creamy smooth. As a gourmet option, serve soup with a spoonful of basil pesto (on page 254) swirled into each bowl. Garnish each bowl with a fresh stem of basil leaves.

Almond Cream

1 cup raw almonds, blanched
1 cup water

In a blender, combine almonds and water and blend on high speed until creamy smooth.

ROASTED RED PEPPER BEAN SOUP
Level One

Summer

A wonderful combination of taste and texture, red bell peppers, with their bell-shaped glossy exterior, are the Christmas ornaments of the plant kingdom. Although red bell peppers are available throughout the year, they are at their peak of taste and are the most abundant during the months of August and September.

3 red bell peppers, cut into halves, seeded and sliced lengthwise into 1/4" strips
1 whole garlic bulb
1 large yellow onion, chopped
4 tablespoons olive oil
2 15-ounce cans organic Cannellini beans, drained and rinsed
1 32-ounce box vegetable broth
1 teaspoon chili peppers
2 teaspoons salt

Preheat oven to 250 degrees. Place red bell peppers and whole garlic bulb on a baking sheet; rub with olive oil and cook for 1 hour, or until peppers are tender. Remove from oven, set the garlic bulb aside; place peppers on a chop block, then chop. In a large skillet, lightly sauté the onion in olive oil for 10 minutes, or until onion is translucent. Remove garlic cloves from bulb. Add peppers and garlic cloves, then sauté for 2-3 more minutes. Add beans, vegetable broth, chili peppers and salt, stirring for 1 minute. Cover and cook for 15 minutes on low heat. Transfer to blender and blend on high speed until creamy smooth. Return to pot, then cover and let sit for 30 minutes.

POTATO CORN SOUP
Level One

Summer – Autumn

Did you know that corn is produced on every continent of the world with the exception of Antarctica? Corn has actually become America's number one field crop. While corn is available in the United States from October through June, its peak season is June, July and August. When combined with potatoes, you'll find that they make the most perfect match!

1 1/2 quarts water
4 cups yellow onion, chopped
3 cups celery, chopped
6 garlic cloves, peeled and minced
2 tablespoons Nama Shoyu Unpasteurized Soy Sauce
5 cups corn kernels, cut off cob
5 cups potatoes, cut into 1-inch cubes
2 tablespoons dill weed
2 teaspoons salt
1/4 teaspoon black pepper
1 tablespoon Organic Earth Balance

In a large soup pot, combine water, onion and celery. Cover and cook on low heat for approximately 20 minutes. Stir in garlic and soy sauce; add corn and potatoes, then cook for another 10 minutes. Remove from heat. Place one-half corn and potato mixture in blender and blend on high speed until creamy smooth. Add dill weed, salt, pepper and Organic Earth Balance, then pulse 3-4 times. Pour purée back into soup pot and stir with remaining soup mixture. Cover and let sit for at least 1 hour.

CREAM OF SHITAKE SOUP
Level One
❖ ❖ ❖ ❖
Anytime

Aside from being top choice for your sauté pan, the healthful benefits of eating shitake mushrooms make them an even more taste treat to marvel over. Deeply rooted in Asian history, the first mention of the shitake dates back to 199 AD, when natives of Kyushu presented the Emperor with a gift of this prized woodland delicacy. During the Ming Dynasty (1368-1644), this mushroom was considered the elixir of life. It was reserved and enjoyed only by the emperor and his family.

5 cups shitake mushrooms, chopped
10 shallots, cut in half and sliced
12 garlic cloves, peeled and minced
2 tablespoons olive oil
1 quart water
2 tablespoons Nama Shoyu Unpasteurized Soy Sauce
1/2 cup red miso

In a large soup pot, sauté mushrooms, shallots, and garlic in olive oil for 10-15 minutes, or until mushrooms are tender. In a blender, combine water, soy sauce and miso and blend on medium speed until creamy smooth; add to soup pot, then stir. Cover and cook for 15-20 minutes. Remove from heat. Add almond cream to soup pot, stir and cover. Allow soup to sit for about 1 hour before serving.

Almond Cream

1 cup almonds, blanched
1 cups water

In a blender, blend almonds and water at high speed until creamy smooth.

CREAMY KALE POTATO SOUP
Level One
❖ ❖ ❖ ❖
Anytime

Kale is a hearty green leafy vegetable that belongs to the Brassica family, a group of vegetables that includes cabbage, collards and Brussels sprouts. Kale gained its widespread attention because of its abundant health-promoting phytonutrients. While kale prefers the cold weather, if cared for correctly, it can produce a surplus of leaves throughout every season, including the winter.

3 cups water
2 cups onions, sliced
2 cups celery, diced
6 garlic cloves, peeled and diced
2 tablespoons Nama Shoyu Unpasteurized Soy Sauce
6 small russet potatoes, cut into bite-size cubes
1 bunch kale, stemmed and thinly diced
2 tablespoons olive oil
1/4 teaspoon salt

In a large soup pot, combine water, onion, celery, garlic and soy sauce and cook on low heat for 15-20 minutes. Transfer to blender and blend on high speed until creamy smooth. Return to pot, then add uncooked potatoes. Cover and cook on low heat for 5 minutes, then stir in kale. Cover and cook on low heat for an additional 10-15 minutes. Remove from heat. Stir in the olive oil and salt. Cover and let sit for 1 hour before serving.

LIMA BEAN SPINACH SOUP
Level One
✣ ✣ ✣ ✣
Anytime

The cultivation of Lima beans spread to North America from the mountainous region of the Andes in the early 1300s. It was during the Spanish Viceroyalty of Peru that lima beans began to be exported to the rest of the Americas and Europe. Because the shipment of Limas had their place of origin in Lima, Peru, the beans got named as such. The interesting thing is that this bean is the only legume on the alkalizing food chain.

2 quarts water
1 quart lima beans, soaked overnight
4 cups yellow onions, diced
12 bay leaves
2 bunches spinach, stemmed and chopped
3 cups tomatoes, diced
8 garlic cloves, peeled and minced
1/4 cup Nama Shoyu Unpasteurized Soy Sauce
1 1/2 tablespoons salt

In a large soup pot, bring water to a slow boil. Reduce heat, then add soaked beans, onion and bay leaves. Cover and cook on low heat for approximately 1 hour, or until beans are soft. Stir in spinach, tomatoes, garlic, soy sauce and salt. Cover and cook for another 10-15 minutes. Remove from heat and let sit for 1 hour before serving.

CREAM OF BROCCOLI SOUP

Level One

✤✤✤✤

Anytime

Simple and delicious, this soup has been a favorite of most everyone for eons, withstanding the taste of time. And the best thing is, you don't even need to add heavy cream to take it to the culinary heights of 5-star gourmet.

5 cups water
2 large yellow onions, chopped
1 large bunch broccoli, chopped
2 tablespoons Nama Shoyu Unpasteurized Soy Sauce
3 tablespoons tarragon
Salt to taste

In a large soup pot, add water, onions, broccoli, soy sauce, tarragon and salt. Cover and cook over low heat for approximately 15 minutes. Transfer to blender and blend on high speed until creamy smooth. Add desired amount of Plum Good Cashew Cream and blend on low speed until well blended. And it really is, plum good!

Plum Good Cashew Cream

1 cup raw cashews
1 cup water
2 tablespoons Ume Plum Vinegar
1 teaspoon salt

In a blender, combine cashews, water, vinegar and salt and blend on high speed until creamy smooth.

ROSEMARY POTATO SOUP
Level One
✤ ✤ ✤ ✤
Anytime

Rosemary is a woody, perennial herb with fragrant evergreen needle-like leaves. Native to the Mediterranean region and member of the mint family, its name is derived from the Latin name rosmarinus, which literally means dew of the sea.

4 cups water
4 cups yellow onions, diced
5 cups squash, sliced
5 garlic cloves, peeled
1/4 cup rosemary, stemmed
3 tablespoons Nama Shoyu Unpasteurized Soy Sauce
5 cups Yukon Gold potatoes, cut into small cubes
1 tablespoon olive oil
2 tablespoons Organic Earth Balance
1 dash cayenne pepper
1 tablespoon salt

In a large soup pot, add water, onions, squash, garlic, rosemary and soy sauce. Cover and cook over a low heat for approximately 15 minutes. Place cubed potatoes in a separate steamer pan; cover and cook for approximately 10 minutes, or until potatoes are soft. Remove from heat. Toss potatoes with olive oil and salt. In a blender, purée soup with Organic Earth Balance, cayenne pepper and salt. Pour into soup pot; add potatoes, cover and let sit for 1 hour.

BLACK BEAN SOUP
Level One

Anytime

Black beans are especially popular in Latin American cuisine. High in protein, magnesium, manganese, folate, potassium, calcium and iron, they are available throughout the year. No matter if they're dried or canned, these beans could not be more descriptively named; they are commonly referred to as turtle beans, most likely because of their shiny, dark, shell-like appearance.

2 cans organic black beans, drained and rinsed

1 large yellow onion, chopped

2 garlic cloves, peeled and chopped

1-2 carrots, peeled and diced

1 teaspoon salt

1 jalapeño pepper, cut in half, seeded and minced

1 teaspoon ground cumin

1/2 teaspoon each dried oregano and thyme

1-32 ounce box vegetable broth

2 tablespoons Nama Shoyu Unpasteurized Soy Sauce

1 avocado, cut in half, pitted, cut into cubes and spooned out

1 cup spring onions, chopped

1 cup fresh cilantro leaves, stemmed and chopped

In a large soup pot, lightly sauté the onion and garlic on low heat in olive oil for 10 minutes, or until onion is translucent. Add carrots, salt, jalapeño pepper, cumin, oregano, and thyme. Sauté for 2-3 more minutes; add vegetable broth and beans. Cover and cook on low heat for 30 minutes. Remove from heat. Add 1/2 cup cilantro, soy sauce, and let sit for 30 minutes. Garnish with chopped spring onions, cilantro and avocado. Delicious served with homemade cornbread.

SWEET POTATO PEA SOUP
Level One

Autumn – Winter

Sweet potatoes and peas go together like two peas in a pod. This recipe was inspired by a soup I was eating one rock-and-roll sunny afternoon at a restaurant called Follow Your Heart in Woodland Hills, Ca. It was 1994, and as I was scraping the last morsel of soup with my spoon, "I felt the earth move under my feet!" At first I thought it was my reaction to the last bite of soup, but then I realized it was an earthquake, and a big one too. My friend and I ducked for shelter under our table like two kids in a school drill. What an experience that was! So if you're ready for a taste shattering experience, let's rock-and-roll!

6 cups water

4 bay leaves

2 cups celery, chopped

3 cups yellow onion, chopped

4 garlic cloves, peeled and pressed

1 tablespoon Nama Shoyu Unpasteurized Soy Sauce

2 cups carrots, peeled and diced

5 cups sweet potatoes, peeled and diced

1 tablespoon Spike seasoning

2 teaspoons dried tarragon

2 teaspoons dried oregano

1 teaspoon dried basil

1/8 teaspoon cayenne pepper

1 10-ounce package Cascadian Farm Organic Frozen Peas

In a large soup pot, add water, bay leaves, celery, onion, garlic and soy sauce. Cook on low heat for 20 minutes. Add carrots, sweet potatoes, Spike seasoning, herbs and cayenne pepper; cover and cook on low heat for 30 minutes. Remove bay leaves. Stir in peas; cover and cook for 10 minutes. In a blender, purée 1/2 soup mixture on high speed; return to soup pot, then stir with reserved soup.

WATERCRESS PEA PUREE
Level One
❋ ❋ ❋ ❋
Autumn – Winter

This warming purée is great on a chilly autumn or wintry day. Snuggled up with a loved one by a fire or served at a dinner party, it's one of those absolutely simple yet gourmet taste delights.

1 quart water
2 bunches watercress, stemmed
2 10-ounce packages Cascadian Farm Organic Frozen Peas
2 tablespoons Organic Earth Balance
1 pinch cayenne pepper
Salt to taste

In a medium-size soup pot, add water and bring to a low boil. Reduce heat to lowest temperature. Add the watercress and peas. Cover and cook for about 15 minutes, or until the peas and watercress are tender. Transfer to a blender; add Organic Earth Balance, cayenne pepper and salt, then blend until creamy smooth.

CREAM OF FENNEL SOUP
Level One

Autumn – Winter

I love to travel. I especially like traveling to various healing centers around the world, curious as to their method of restoring a healthy balance back to an unhealthy terrain. This recipe was inspired by one of the soups I had in Switzerland while visiting Dr. Rau's famous Paracelsus Clinic. Dr. Rau's health diet consisted of a fare of mostly soups and salads. This soup was one of my favorites.

2 quarts water
5 russet potatoes, 3 unpeeled and diced,
  and 2 peeled and diced
2 fennel bulbs, chopped
1 medium onion, chopped
2 tablespoons fresh dill
1 dash cayenne pepper
1 tablespoon Organic Earth Balance
1 tablespoon Nama Shoyu Unpasteurized Soy Sauce
1 tablespoon salt

In a steamer pan, steam the 3 unpeeled diced potatoes on low heat for 10 minutes. In a large soup pot, bring the water to a slow boil. Reduce heat to lowest temperature. Add the steamed potatoes, fennel and onion and cook for approximately 15 minutes. Transfer to blender; add dill, cayenne pepper, Organic Earth Balance, soy sauce and salt and blend on high speed until creamy smooth. Steam the 2 remaining peeled diced potatoes for 10 minutes. Return puréed soup to soup pot; add the 2 steamed peeled potatoes and stir. Cover and let sit for 1 hour.

SWEET POTATO COCONUT SOUP
Level One

Autumn

Sweet potatoes and coconut milk make the perfect counterpart for this wintry, gingery soup. All you have to do is peel, open and shake and there you have it. Not only is it easy to make, it's simply delicious.

1 quart water

5 sweet potatoes, peeled and sliced

1" chunk fresh ginger, sliced

1 13.5-ounce can organic coconut milk

3 tablespoons Nama Shoyu Unpasteurized Soy Sauce

2 tablespoons coconut oil

1 teaspoon crushed red pepper flakes

1 teaspoon salt

In a medium-size soup pot, add water, sweet potatoes (if desired, yams can be substituted for sweet potatoes) and ginger. Cover and cook over low heat for 10-15 minutes, or until sweet potatoes are tender. Stir in coconut milk, soy sauce, coconut oil, salt, and crushed red pepper flakes. Remove from heat. Cover and let sit for 30 minutes. Transfer to blender and blend on high speed until creamy smooth. Delicious served with one scoop of organic jasmine rice.

CREAM OF CARROT SAGE SOUP
Level One

Autumn – Winter

As a medicinal herb, sage steps up to the plate. The Latin name for sage is salvia, which means to heal. During the Middle Ages, sage was often used as medicine. The motto was, Cur moriatur homo cul Salvia crescit in horto, which means why should a man die while sage grows in his garden? Good point. Overtime, sage grew to be a culinary favorite. It now holds center stage during our two most festive holidays, Thanksgiving and Christmas.

3 cups water
3 1/2 cups carrots, peeled and sliced
1 medium yellow onion, diced
3 large garlic cloves, peeled and minced
1/2 cup fresh sage, chopped
2 tablespoons Nama Shoyu Unpasteurized Soy Sauce
1/8 teaspoon cayenne pepper
1 1/2 teaspoon salt

In a medium-size soup pot, bring water to a low boil. Turn down heat to lowest temperature. Add carrots, onion and garlic. Cover and cook for approximately 15-20 minutes. Remove from heat. Transfer to a blender, then add the sage, soy sauce, cayenne pepper and salt and blend on high speed until creamy smooth. Pour back into pan; add 1 cup cashew cream and swirl. When ready to serve, drizzle the remaining cashew cream along with a touch of olive oil over the top.

Cashew Cream

1 cup raw cashews
1 cup water

In a blender, combine cashews and water and blend on high speed until creamy smooth.

VEGETABLE BEAN CHILI
Level One

Winter

While the country of origin for chili is Mexico, it didn't take long for the aroma of chili con carne to ride the air stream north and become the official dish of Texas. While traditional chili is made with chopped or ground beef, this vegetarian version was a favorite of most every customer who walked through the doors of my vegetarian restaurant.

2 16-ounce cans ground organic tomatoes

3 cups water

3 medium yellow onions, cut into bite size pieces

4 carrots, peeled, and diced

1 large red, 1 green and 1 yellow bell pepper

1 tablespoon chili peppers

2-3 tablespoons chili powder

3 cans pinto beans

2 tablespoons olive oil

2 1/2 tablespoons salt

In a large soup pot, combine tomatoes, water, onions and carrots and cook on low heat for 10 minutes. Add bell peppers, chili peppers and chili powder, then stir. Cook for another 10 minutes. Remove from heat. Add beans, olive oil and salt. Cover and let sit for approximately 1 hour.

CREAM OF BRUSSELS SPROUTS SOUP
Level One

Autumn – Winter

Production of Brussels sprouts in the United States began around 1800 when French settlers brought them to Louisiana. They soon found their way to the California's central coast, which offered them an ideal combination of coastal fog and cool temperatures year-round; the harvest season lasts from June to January. This soup is an absolute dinner party favorite!

4 cups Brussels sprouts
2 cups water
1 small yellow onion, chopped
1/8 cup tarragon
1/8 cup organic capers
1 tablespoon Nama Shoyu Unpasteurized Soy Sauce
1 teaspoon salt

In a medium-size soup pot, combine Brussels sprouts, water, yellow onion and tarragon and cook over low heat for 10-15 minutes, or until Brussels sprouts are soft. Add soy sauce and salt, then stir. Transfer to a blender and blend on high speed until blended. Add cashew cream and blend again on low speed, then transfer to a serving bowl and garnish with tarragon twigs.

Cashew Cream

1/2 cup raw cashews
1/2 cup water

In a blender, combine cashews and water and blend on high speed until creamy smooth.

GAZPACHO AVOCADO SOUP
Level One & Two

Summer

Even though this soup originated from the southern Spanish region of Andalusia, it didn't take long for it to become an Italian and French tradition. Families of all ages come together in the afternoons in their small village piazzas to enjoy this healthy-heart-filled bowl of tomato heaven. Although there are many regional and modern-day versions, this is my favorite one of all! Join me, won't you?

3 vine-ripe tomatoes, cut in half

1 cucumber, peeled, cut in half, seeded and chopped

1 green bell pepper, cut in half, seeded and chopped

1/2 red onion, peeled, quartered and thinly sliced

2 garlic cloves, peeled and minced

1 cup parsley, stemmed and finely chopped

1 jalapeño pepper, cut in half, seeded and minced

3 tablespoons red wine vinegar

1/4 cup olive oil

1 teaspoon salt

2 avocados, halved, pitted, cut into cubes and spooned out

Using a food processor or blender, pulse the tomatoes, cucumbers, bell peppers, onions, garlic, parsley, jalapeño pepper, vinegar, olive oil and salt 3-4 times, or until finely chopped. Transfer to a large bowl and add avocado as a delicious, but very untraditional, bite-size garnish.

RAW CUCUMBER DILL SOUP
Level One & Two

Spring – Summer

The cucumber is believed to have originated in India. Evidence also indicates that it has been cultivated in Western Asia for 3,000 years. As a natural diuretic, it is used in the fitness world by bodybuilders and people trying to lose weight. Combined with dill weed, it is scrumptiously delicious.

1 large cucumber, peeled

1 tablespoon coconut oil

1 clove garlic, peeled

1 small cayenne pepper, cut in half & deseed

1 tablespoon dill weed, fresh or dried

1 small red bell pepper, deseeded and finely chopped

1/2 teaspoon salt

1/2 cup edible flowers

Using a blender or food processor, purée the cucumber, coconut oil, garlic, cayenne pepper and dill weed at high speed until smooth. Transfer to a large serving bowl. Stir in the bell peppers and season with salt. Serve cold and garnish with edible flower and/or a sprig of dill weed.

RAW TOMATO BASIL SOUP
Level One & Two
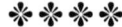
Summer

This recipe is a great summer alternative to the traditional hot tomato basil soup served even in the finest of gourmet restaurants. Basil is originally native to Iran and India and other tropical regions of Asia, having been cultivated there for more than 5,000 years. The word basil comes from the Greek word basileus, which means king, and is believed to have grown above the spot where St. Constantine and Helen discovered the Holy Cross. There are speculations that basil may have even been used as a healing ointment in royal baths. In my culinary experience, it definitely goes down as the tastiest king of herbs.

6 vine-ripened tomatoes, cut in half

1 cup basil leaves, chopped

1/2 cup yellow onion, chopped

1 celery stalk, chopped

1 avocado, cut in half, pitted, cut into cubes and spooned out

1/4 cup olive oil

1 tablespoon Nama Shoyu Unpasteurized Soy Sauce

1 dash cayenne pepper

1 teaspoon salt

1 lime, juiced

Using a food processor or blender, pulse 3-4 times, or until chunky-smooth. Transfer to a large serving bowl and garnish with basil leaves.

PINEAPPLE GAZPACHO SOUP
Level One & Two

Summer

This sweet tropical fruit is a favorite for all ages. Pineapples contain bromelain, an enzyme that holds the key to many of pineapple's health benefits.

4 cups pineapple, chopped
4 cups cucumber, peeled & chopped
3-4 tablespoons jalapeño peppers, minced
4 tablespoons scallions, thinly sliced mostly white part
2 tablespoons lime juice
1 cup fresh pineapple juice
1 teaspoon salt (optional)
1 cup cilantro leaves
1 avocado, seeded and chopped

Using a blender or food processer, purée 3 cups pineapple, 3 cups cucumber, jalapeño peppers, scallions, lime juice, pineapple juice, and salt. Add the remaining pineapple and cucumber and cilantro. Pulse the blender quickly a few times—the gazpacho should remain chunky. Stir in the avocado. Delicious!

SPROUTED BEAN CHILI
Level One & Two

Spring – Summer – Autumn

For those who love chili but desire a more raw food fare, this one's for you!

5 tomatoes
2 avocadoes
1/2-cup sun-dried tomatoes
2 teaspoons salt
2 teaspoons cumin
1 tablespoon chili peppers
2 carrots
1 celery stalk
2 leeks
1 red bell pepper
1 yellow bell pepper
1/4-cup olive oil
1 cup sprouted mung beans

Using a blender or food processor, blend tomatoes, avocado, sun-dried tomatoes, salt, cumin, chili peppers in blender. Chop vegetables into small cubes, place in a glass bowl, massage with olive oil and salt, and marinate for several hours. Mix all ingredients and serve with dehydrated crackers.

REFERENCE NOTES

Introduction: Insights from the Author

For insights into global warming, I have referred to Al Gore's book and film, *An Inconvenient Truth: The Crisis of Global Warming*, revised edition (New York: Viking, 2007); and www.climatecrisis.net, the official site for the film *An Inconvenient Truth*, featuring Al Gore (Paramount, 100 min., 2006).

See Ann Wigmore, *The Hippocrates Diet and Health Program: A Natural Diet and Health Program for Weight Control, Disease Prevention, and Life Extension* (Avery, imprint of Penguin Group USA, 1984) for the medical philosophy of Hippocrates (460-377 B.C.E).

For the description of the lives of Béchamp and Pasteur and their contrasting theories, I referred to Nancy Appleton's book, *The Curse of Louis Pasteur: Why Medicine Is Not Healing a Diseased World* (Santa Monica: Choice Publishing, 1999).

For an introduction to the internal terrain theory and the amazing habits of microzymas, I referred to Christopher Bird's book, "To Be or Not to Be? 150 Years of Hidden Knowledge" *(Nexus,* April 1992).

Part One
Chapter One: What is an EcoDiet?

In writing this chapter, I explain the meaning of an EcoDiet, what a diet really means and what eco really means. To set the stage for the rest of the book, I have also defined ecosystems and the hierarchy of the food chain.

Chapter Two: Dietary Devolution

Dietary Devolution #1 – Cardiologist William C. Roberts, editor in chief of *The American Journal of Cardiology* and medical director of the Baylor Heart and Vascular Institute at Baylor University Medical Center in Dallas, is cited in Sally Deneen, "Body of Evidence: Were Humans Meant to Eat Meat?" *E/The Environmental Magazine*, vol. XIII, no. 1 (Jan/Febr 2002), www.emagazine.com

Milton R. Mills, M.D., is associate director of preventative medicine for the *Physicians Committee for Responsible Medicine* (PCRM) based in Washington, D.C. His article "The Comparative Anatomy of Eating," with the accompanying chart, can be found at www.vegsource.com/veg_faq/comparative.htm

For research pertaining to the different effects of acid animal proteins versus alkaline plant proteins, refer to the studies of Deborah E. Sellmeyer, Katie L. Stone, Anthony Sebastian, Steven R. Cummings and for the Study of Osteoporotic Fractures Research Group, UNC-SF, "A High Ratio of Dietary Animal to Vegetable Protein Increases the Rate of Bone Loss and the Risk of Fracture in Postmenopausal Women," American Journal of Clinical Nutrition 73, no. 1 (January 2001): 118-122; and Anthony Sebastian, Lynda A. Frassetto, Deborah E. Sellmeyer, Renée L. Merriam and R. Curtis Morris, Jr., "Estimation of the Net Acid Load of the Diet of Ancestral Preagricultural Homo Sapiens and their Hominid Ancestors," American Journal of Clinical Nutrition 76, no. 6 (December 2002): 1308-1316.

See T. Colin Campbell, Ph.D, with Thomas M. Campbell II, *The China Study: Startling Implications for Diet, Weight Loss and Long-term Health* (Dallas, TX: BenBella Books, 2004), introduction; and Marla Cone, "Ancestral Diet Gone Toxic," *Los Angeles Times,* January 13, 2004, A-1, also at http://articles.latimes.com/2004/jan/13/local/me-inuit13

Red-meat Diet Ups Odds of Earth Death, *The Virginia-Pilot and The Ledger-Star, Norfolk, VA, March 24, 2009.*

A 2006 United Nations report: H. Steinfeld et al., Livestock's Long Shadow: Environmental Issues and Options, Livestock, Environment and Development (2006).

Dietary Devolution #2 – The Hunters of the Arctic: bambusspiele.de. Retrieved on 2008-01-07. http://alaska.usgs.gov/science/biology/p
Sources on biomagnification: http://users.rcn.com/jkimball.ma.ultrane
http://www.marietta.edu/~biol/102/2bioma
http://www.ncbi.nlm.nih.gov/pubmed/16986
http://www.ehjournal.net/content/6/1/32

Toxic Fish – Source: Associated Content *Information from the source.*http://www.associatedcontent.com/article/7898

Factory-farmed Animals: Animals Raised In Factory Farms – Antibiotics: Farm sanctuary – rescue – education – advocacy www.factoryfarming.com

Mad Cow Disease – Source: Wikipedia Encyclopedia: wikipedia.org., World Health Organization (WHO) avian influenza website.

Wikipedia Encyclopedia: Compassion in World Farming – Environment & sustainability

Chemical Agriculture: soil pollution – www.pollutionissues.com/re-sy/soil-pollution.html

Robert Buist, *Food Chemical Sensitivity: What It Is and How to Cope with It* (Garden City Park, N.Y., Avery Pub. Group, 1986).

Paula Baillie-Hamilton, M.D., Ph.D., *The Body Restoration Plan: Eliminate Chemical Calories and Repair Your Body's Natural Slimming System* (Shaklee Corporation, 2002). This is a little-known, but truly valuable, resource.

U.S. Department of Agriculture, Economic Research Service, "U.S. Fertilizer Use and Price." September 25, 2006 (accessed October 13, 2006).

Food Irradiation – Source: State of our Food

www.healthgoods.com/education/nutrition

Genetically Modified Food – Source: Mothers for Natural Law; http://www.safe-food.org/-issue/dangers.html – Washington Times, March 11, 1997; Village Voice, March 10, 1998. "The End of Nature – From Banana Vaccines to Fast-Growing Fish: DNA Let Scientists Play God" by Mark Schoofs.

Dietary Devolution #3 – Source: Convenience Foods Save Little Time, Lack Nutrients, Judith Groch, Senior Writer, MedPage Today, http:www.medpagetoday.com/PrimaryCare/DietNutrition/dh/6368

Source: All the Health Risks of Processed Foods – In Just a Few Quick, Convenient Bites, SixWise.com, http://www.sixwise.com/newsletters/05/10/19/all_the_health_risks_of MSG: For more information about the truth of MSG, see the Wikipedia Encyclopedia

Aspartame: Source – Janet Starr Hull, Creator of the Aspartame Detox Program http://www.sweetpoison.com/aspartame-information.html

Information about the exposure of toxic chemicals in fast food milkshakes can be found on Dr. Joseph Mercola's blog, http://blogs.mercola.com/sites/vitalvotes/archive/2007/07/09/Fast-Food   Milkshakes-Exposed.aspx

Chapter Three: The Power of pH

In writing this chapter, I have often relied on the superlative wisdom and clarity of Dr. M. T. Morter, Jr. as it regards to pH and the acid-alkaline balance. I've especially gleaned a lot of my knowledge of pH and the human body from his volume *Correlative Urinalysis: The Body Knows Best* (Rogers, AR: B.E.S.T. Research Inc. 1987). Dr. Morter is a great researcher, teacher, and mentor, whose understanding of the body and the ramifications of the acid-alkaline balance never cease to amaze me. For a general guide into this subject, see Dr. Morter's *Your Health, Your Choice: Your Complete Personal Guide to Wellness, Nutrition & Disease Prevention* (Hollywood, FL: Fell Publishers, 1990).

For the table of elements in the human body, see H. A. Harper, V. W. Rodwell, P. A. Mayes, *Review of Physiological Chemistry,* 16th ed. (Los Altos, CA: Lange Medical Publications, 1977).

Bodies of Water and Chemical Pollution: Source: Peter Montague – "Pollution of World's Largest Lakes Shows Importance of Banning Toxics," The Environmental Research Foundation publication 146 (September 11, 1989), www.rachel.org.

Doug Jeanneret, "Lake Erie Water Quality: Past, Present and Future," Fact Sheet 046 (Columbus, OH: Ohio Sea Grant College Program, 1989), and others at http://ohioseagrant. osu.edu.

Candida and the over consumption of fat research can be found in Dr. Doug Graham's book, *The 80-10-10 Diet.*

Dr. Tullio Simoncini, M.D., *Cancer is a Fungus* (Rome, Italy: Edizioni Lampis, 2007), http://www.cancerisafungus.com.

Otto Warburg, "The Prime Cause and Prevention of Cancer," translated and edited by Dean Burk, National Cancer Institute (Lecture delivered to Nobel Laureates at Lindau, by Lake

Constance, Germany, on June 30, 1966). Otto Warburg was the director of the Max Planck Institute for Cell Physiology, Berlin, Germany. He was the recipient of two Nobel Prizes and many other awards and honors for his work in the chemistry and physics of life. Retrieved from www.ozonetherapy.co.uk

Otto Warburg, The Prime Cause and Prevention of Cancer, 1966, pg.6.

Dr. Sam Whang, *Reverse Aging* (JSP Publishing, 1991). Sang Whang, founder of AlkaLife International, is an engineer, scientist and inventor with many U.S. patents.

For more updated biographical information on Max Planck, see: Planck, Max, Scientific Autobiography and Other Papers. Philosophical Library, New York, 1949.

Dr. Koch, M.D., Ph.D., a graduate of the University of Michigan, a well-published pathologist and medical school professor. Source: Diamond WJ, *et al.* An alternative medicine definitive guide to cancer. Tiburon, California: Future Medicine Publishing, Inc., 1997:34,922.

Quotes: William Howard Hay, M.D., was a New York doctor, author, lecturer and founder of The East Aurora Sun and Diet Sanatorium. A traditional physician for the first 16 years of his career, this New York doctor introduced the world to food combining, ran a successful sanatorium for many years and was a renowned lecturer on health topics. After curing himself from Bright's disease through proper diet, he wrote several books including, *A New Health Era* (1939). See the Wikipedia

Chapter Four: Internal Acid Rain

The Harmful Effects Of Acid Rain: See U.S. EPA (Environmental Protection Agency) website, http://www.epa.gov/acidrain, for a basic overview of acid rain and its effects.

Internal Acid Rain and Neurological Diseases: For more information on metabolism as it pertains to coenzymes and oxidation, see *Exercise Physiology – Energy, Nutrition, & Human Performance*, Chapter 5, page 131, by author William D. McArdle.

Quote: Dr. Lorne Label is associate clinical professor of neurology at the David Geffen School of Medicine at UCLA, adjunct faculty at Loyola Marymount University, medical director of both the Southern California Attention Deficit Disorder Clinic and the Brain Longevity Center, and is in private practice with California Neurological Specialists, where he practices adult and pediatric neurology and medical acupuncture.

Quote: Rudolph Virchow (1821-1902) was a German medical scientist and politician. He founded the medical disciplines of cellular pathology and comparative pathology. He was also among the early founders of anthropology and a fervent advocate of democracy at a time when such ideas were considered revolutionary.

Chapter Five: Internal Acid Rain Study
For more information on pH, electrolytes and buffering, see Dr. Ted Morter's books, *Your Health, Your Choice: Your Complete Personal Guide to Wellness, Nutrition & Disease Prevention* (Hollywood, FL: Fell Publishers, 1990), and *Correlative Urinalysis: The Body Knows Best* (Rogers, AR: B.E.S.T. Research, Inc. 1987).

Chapter Six: Stop Acidifying…And Start Alkalizing!
Quote: The U.S. Department of Health ranking of America www.sharpweblabs.com

The Wrong and Right Kind of Salt – For more information on the wrong kind of salt and the health benefits of the right kind of salt, such as the Celtic Sea Salt, refer to studies reported by Selina at the Celtic Sea Salt Company, Asheville, NC.

The Wrong and Right Kind of Oil – The overall information in this section on the wrong kind of oil and the health benefits of the right kind of oil was condensed from the writings of Dr. Udo Erasmus, renowned authority on fats and human nutrition and author of *Choosing the Right Fats*. For more information, you can also refer to his website at www.udosoil.com

Trans-fats–Harvard School of Public Health press release, "Harvard Review of Evidence Verifies that Eating *Trans* Fats Increases Risk of Heart Disease," June 23, 1999, http://www.hsph.harvard.edu/news/press-releases/archives/1999-releases press06231999.html

The Wrong and Right Kind of Sugar – Information on the wrong kind of sugar and the health benefits of consuming the right kind of sugar was obtained from the Wikipedia Encyclopedia and articles published by the Weston Price Foundation. Weston Price Foundation: *Double Dangers of High Fructose* Corn Syrup; http://www.westonaprice.org/modernfood/highfructose.html

From Wikipedia Encyclopedia: Marshall et al. (1957). "Enzymatic Conversion of d-Glucose to d-Fructose." *Science* 125 (3249): 648. Doi: 10.1126/science.125.3249.648. PMID 13421660.

The journal, *Environmental Health* in 2009, reported that high fructose corn syrup was commonly tainted with mercury: www.ehjournal.net/content/8/1/2. McKinney, Matt. of the *Star Tribune:* Minneapolis, St. Paul, Minnesota, January 26, 2009 reported a study conducted by the Institute for Agriculture and Trade Policy, a nonprofit group based in Minneapolis, that trace amounts of mercury were found in processed foods; group says high fructose corn syrup to blame.

Stop Acidifying!
Strong Acid-Forming Foods & Drinks
Animal meat and their byproducts – correlative Urinalysis: The Body Knows Best; Dr. M.T. Morter, Jr. page 80.

Processed Meats: Nitrites and Nitrates: Source Kross, B.C., G.R Hallberg, D.R. Bruner, K. Cherryholmes, and J.K. Johnson (1993) The Nitrate Contamination of Private Well Water in Iowa. Am J Public Health 83:270-272.

Bruning-Fann, C.S., J.B. Kaneene (1993) The effects of nitrate, nitrite, and N-nitroso compounds on human health: a review. Vet Human Toxicology 35:521-538.

Organic Animal Farming: Grass-fed organic meats: Sources: *J Animal Sci 80(5): 1202-11, 2002*; File CLA – Eat Organic Meat

Factory-Farmed Animals & Processed Meats: "Comparing Organic and Intensive Meat Farming Methods," web-page article, http://www.organic-food-for-everyone.co.uk/meat-farming.html/ Chickens & Egg farms – egg industry report: www.eggindustry.com

Pasteurized dairy products: Organic Pastures; Dr. William Campbell Douglass II, M.D., "The Raw Truth about Real Milk," *The Douglass Report,* 2008, http://www.douglassreport.com/reports/raw-milk.pdf

Lactose intolerance - A 2006 human study published in the *Journal of Allergy and Clinical Immunology* on humans and raw milk was obtained from the Weston Price Foundation at: www.westonaprice.org/rawmilk/

Farm-raised fish: Study finds farm-raised salmon laden with cancer-causing chemicals; *Philadelphia Inquirer* (January 9, 2004), found at http://www.organicconsumers.org/

Ken Cook, "Mercury in Your Fish," 2001, http://articles.mercola.com/sites/articles/archive/2001/04/25/mercury-fish-part-one.aspx

Non-Toxic Seafood: Information on safe fish was compiled from Environment, Health and Safety Online at http://www.ehso.com/ehshome/pfiesteria.htm

Drinks: Dr. Anthony von Fraunhofer's study (*General Dentistry,* July/August 2004) on the effects of soft drinks on tooth enamel has been widely reported. See for example, Stan Diel, "Energy Drinks Are 10 Times Worse For Teeth Than Colas" (May 2, 2008), on the WorldDental.org website. See also Pamela R.Erickson, D.D.S.,Deanna L.Alevizos, D.D.S., and Darcy J.Rindelaub, D.D.S. "Soft Drinks: Hard on Teeth," Clinical Feature, *Northwest Dentistry* (March-April 2001), http://www.mndental.org/client_files/documents/Soft_Drinks_Hard_on_Teeth.pdf. Documentation of mineral losses from the metabolism of soft drinks was reported in R.A.S. Hemat and R. Hemat, Principles of Orthomolecularism (Urotext, 2003).

Carson E. Pierce of the Alkalize for Health Organization, class handout. If someone you know has cancer, you might want to take a look at the website of Alkalize for Health, www.alkalizeforhealth.net/summary.htm.

Plastic Bottled Water: Research on the dangers of bottled water can be found at: http://www.ioniczone.com/Plastic_Bottled_Water_Dangers.php

Mild Acid-Forming Foods & Drinks
Organically-Biodynamically-Grown Foods – Organic-Biodynamic Farming: The Josephine Porter Institute for Applied Biodynamics, Inc.: www.appliedbiodynamics.org

Rudolf Steiner (1861-1925): Anthroposophy. Biographical introduction for farmers; www.biodynamics.com/steiner.html

The difference in nutritional value: The Smith Report – Organic Foods vs Commercial Supermarket Foods: Element Levels by Bob L. Smith; Doctor's Data, Inc.; published in the Journal of Applied Nutrition, Volume 45-1, 1993. Copyright International Academy of Nutrition and Preventive Medicine.

Studies on health disorders resulting from petroleum-based chemicals and pesticides compiled August, 1998 by Richard Pessinger, M.Ed., and Wayne Sinclair, M.D., can be found at www.chem-tox.com. The majority of information at Chem-Tox has been attained from the University of Florida and University of South Florida Medical Libraries.

The effects of simply washing pesticide residue from your foods with soap and water: Paula Baillie-Hamilton, M.D., Ph.D., environmental-health specialist and author of *Toxic Overload* (Avery, 2005).

The Healing Power of Minerals, Special Nutrients and Trace Elements by Paul Bergner (1997, Prima Publishing, Rocklin, CA) includes USDA figures that show a decline in mineral and vitamin content of several fruits and vegetables between 1914, 1963, and 1992. Table 1 is a summary of mineral decreases in fruits and vegetables over a 30-year period, adapted from Bergner's book.

Most commercially-grown grains and beans in the U.S. are produced from hybrid seeds. See the Wikipedia Encyclopedia on hybrid seeds.

In 2004, a study was conducted to evaluate possible changes in USDA nutrient data for 43 garden crops between 1950 and 1999. The report, published in the *Journal of the American College of Nutrition,* Source: Foodbank of North Central Arkansas.
http://www.jacn.org/cgi/content/abstract/23/6/669
http://www.fbnca.org/Heirloom_Seed_Shop.html#hybrid

Quote from Dr. Bernard Jensen; mineral-deficient soil *Empty Harvest* page 8.

Organic produce is healthier than commercially-grown produce: ThisIsLondon.co.uk (Evening Standard) - 10/29/07

Organic Grains & Legumes: Health Benefits of Grains & Beans: *European Journal of Clinical Nutrition* (2006) 60, 1145–1159. doi:10.1038/sj.ejcn.1602435; published online 3 May 2006 - http://www.nature.com/ejcn/journal/v60/n10/abs/1602435a.html

Information on high levels of phytic acid, also known as phytates can be found on in the book: Nourishing Traditions by Sally Fallon, Page 25.

Organic Soy Foods: According to the Weston A. Price Foundation in Washington, D.C.

adverse studies on soy foods can be found at: http://www.westonaprice.org/soy/index.html

From Natural Life Magazine, January/February 2005 Ask Natural Life:
Are Soy Foods Safe? – authored by Wendy Priesnitz.
Fermented Soy Products – Fermentation reduces the phytic acid (phytates) and anti-nutrient levels of soybeans, making their nourishment available to the human digestive system. See the Wikipedia Encyclopedia on Phytic Acid.

Berries: Acids are not the same. A recent study found that resveratrol, a plant phytochemical found in blueberries, strongly inhibited the replication of the influenza virus in cell cultures. http://www.nowfoods.com/?action=itemdetail&item_id=45433&TPL_NAME=printview. tpl resveratrol - Resveratrol: Nature's Flu Vaccine?

Fruits such as cranberries have been found to reduce the risk of heart disease. Most recently, a study presented at the annual congress of the International Union of Physiological Sciences in March/April 2005 found that pigs with atherosclerosis (a primary causes of heart disease) that received a daily dose of cranberry powder had restored blood vessel health. Source: http://healing.about.com/od/recipes/a/cranberries.htm

Start Alkalizing!
Strong Alkaline-Forming Foods & Drinks
Dark Green Leafy Vegetables – Information on the Swedish study can be found at http://www.vegetarian-nutrition.info/updates/benefits-of-green-leafy-vegetables.php

Mild Alkaline-Forming Foods & Drinks
Fruits and Vegetables – Vinson J, Su X, Zubik L, Bose P: Phenol antioxidant quantity and quality in foods: fruits. *J Agric Food Chem* 2001, 49:5315-532

Chapter Seven: The Four "Fuel" Groups
Air – The Alkaline Breath: Conscious Breathing: For information on conscious breathing I have referred to, Andrew Weil, M.D., author of Natural Health, Natural Medicine, who is a world-renowned leader and pioneer in the field of integrative medicine. Dr. Weil is the founder and director of the Arizona Center for Integrative Medicine at the University of Arizona Health Sciences Center, where he is also a Clinical Professor of Medicine and Professor of Public Health and the Lovell-Jones Professor of Integrative Rheumatology. Dr.

Weil received both his medical degree and his undergraduate AB degree in biology (botany) from Harvard University. For more information on conscious breathing, see Dr. Weil's DVD series, *Breathing: The Master Key to Self-Healing* www.drweil.com

Sheldon Saul Hendler, M.D., Ph.D., brings hard core science to the masses through his groundbreaking book, *The Oxygen Breakthrough*. In his book he not only brings us the science behind the power of our breath, he outlines breathing exercises that can transform what some call disease when, in fact, what most suffer from is a lack of oxygen.

Indoor Air Pollution: United States Environmental Protection (EPA) – Regarding documented research on indoor air quality, I referred to articles on site, http://www.epa.gov/iaq/voc.html#Sources

Consumer Product Safety Commission (CPSC) (1992) Labeling requirements for art materials presenting chronic hazards; guidelines for determining chronic toxicity of products subject to the FHSA 16 CFR § 1500.135; See also Federal Register preamble and supplementary definition of "toxic" under the Federal Hazardous Substances Act. 57 Fed. Reg. 46626-46674 (1992).

For more information on toxic indoor air refer to http://www.cpsc.gov/cpscpub/pubs/450.html

Fire – The Alkaline Sun: For information on our relationship to the sun, I referenced, Michael Holick, M.D., Professor of Medicine, Physiology and Biophysics, Director of the General Clinical Research Center, Director of the Bone Health Care Clinic – Boston University Medical Center, and author of *The UV Advantage*. Dr. Holick is the world's foremost authority on vitamin D and the healing power of natural sunlight. For more information about his research on sunlight and vitamin D, visit his website at: www.uvadvantage.org

Exposure to natural sunlight has also been shown to increase the number of white blood cells in the body, which plays the leading role in defending against invasions by bacteria and foreign organisms. http://www.naturalmedicinefordisease.com/Main/Sunshine

Drink Your Sunscreen: Studies that refer to "drinking your sunscreen," submitted by "Avoid Cancer Now" on May 22, 2008; report can be found on http://medheadlines.com/2008/05/22/

eat-your-sunscreen-10-superfoods-to-lower-skin-cancer-risk/

For sunscreen dangers go to:
http://www.worldimagenaturals.com/blog/archives/000026_sunscreen_dangers.html

The Douglas Report: http://www.douglassreport.com/reports/sun/

Sun-Gazing – Studies regarding sun-gazing practices have been reported by India's sun gazer, Hira Ratan Manek who is said to have given himself to NASA for scientific monitoring. It is re further reports that he was able to survive for extended periods solely on light and occasional beverages, water and buttermilk, which he only consumed out of politeness when they were offered. For more information on sun-gazing, visit Hira Ratan Manek's website: http://www.solarhealing.com

For more needed information on sun-gazing, I also referred to the Wikipedia Encyclopedia.

Earth – The Alkaline Foods: Various studies conducted by the Weston A. Price Foundation have been conducted on the subject of the dietary habits and their relationship to the health and longevity of most primitive people and tribal cultures around the globe. These studies can be found at: (1) www.westonaprice.org and (2) http://www.rejoiceinlife.com/mediaFliers/WAPBrochure.php

Eat Raw, Living Foods – Information on the raw food living diet, raw foodist and raw foodism were obtained from the Wikepedia Encyclopedia: (1) "Raw Food Diet – RawGuru.com – Raw Foods – Raw Food Interview." Retrieved on 2008-11-07 (2) "Dietary Lifestyles," Crain, L (2004) www.medhunters.com/articles/dietarylifestylespartfournaturalhygiene.html, and (3) "Raw Food Diet – What is the Raw Food Diet." Altmedicine.about.com Retrieved on 2008-11-07.

Information on enzymes can be found on Page 30 in Dr. Norman Walker's book, *Vibrant Health*.

For more information on how a raw living foods diet can turn both type 1 and 2 diabetes around in 30 days refer to Dr. Gabriel Cousin's DVD, "Raw for 30 Days."

Let's Get Juiced – For more information on juicing, see Dr. Norman Walker's book, *Fresh Vegetable and Fruit Juices*.

Enjoy a Daily Smoothie – Color Me Healthy – Information on the healing power of colors and food can be found at www. pbhfoundation.org

Eat Fermented Foods – For more information on the health benefits of eating fermented foods see Natural Health Publication, Nov, 2007 by Marie Myung Ok Lee.

Eat Locally Grown, Seasonal Foods – Community Supported Agriculture (CSA), visit the website: http://www.localharvest.org/csa

To understand more about the Chinese philosophy on seasonal eating see www.chinadaily.com

Fruits and Vegetables season calendar: Information was compiled from the Third Street Farmer's Market, Santa Monica, California.

Follow the Circadian Rhythm – Refinetti R (2006) *Circadian Physiology, 2nd ed.* CRC Press, Boca Raton. Also referred to Wikipedia Encyclopedia and www.ehow.com/circadianrhythm

Food Combining – For information on food combining, I referred to the father of food combining, Dr. Herbert Shelton and his book *Food Combining Made Easy.*

Mindful Under-eating and Periodic Fasting – Recent studies on under-eating and periodic fasting were conducted at the Laboratory of Neurosciences, National Institute of Aging Gerontology Research Center, Laboratory of Neurosciences and Comparative Medicine, National Institute on Aging, Department of Human Genetics; and Department of Neuroscience and John Hopkins University School of Medicine. They have each reported that both under-eating, due to calorie restrictions and intermittent fasting, with maintained vitamin and mineral intake, can extend lifespan and increase resistance to disease.

Water – The Alkaline Drink: The description of a water molecule: Wikipedia Encyclopedia. For more information on the importance of drinking lots of water every day, F. Batmanghelidj, M.D., author of *Your Body's Many Cries For Water:* says, "You're not sick; you're thirsty. Don't treat thirst with medication."

Drink Ionized Alkaline Water – Ionization: Wikipedia Encyclopedia

Pink, Daniel H. (April 19, 2006). "Investing in Tomorrow's Liquid Gold." Yahoo

West, Larry (March 26, 2006). "World Water Day: A Billion People Worldwide Lack Safe Drinking Water."

Negative health effects of drinking contaminated water, refer to The Center for Disease Control and Prevention (CDC) at, http://www.cdc.gov/

Research on the health benefits of drinking alkaline ionized water can be found in the book, *The Water Puzzle and the Hexagonal Key,* written by researcher Dr. Mu Shik John.

Take a Detox Bath – For more information on the cleansing effects of a 30-minute "Sole" detox bath, refer to the book *Water and Salt – The Essence of Life,* authored by Barbara Hendel.

Colonic Hydrotherapy – The healthful use of colonic hydrotherapy, according to the Royal Society of Medicine, can be found on-line at - *http://www.omx2u.com/articles/colon.asp* and at – The Secret Cause of 90% of all Chronic Diseases, I referred to Dr. Joseph Esposito's article published on June 13, 2007:
http://www.healthsolutions.net/articles/2007/June/digestion/probiotics

Chapter Eight: The Get Clean Go Green EcoDiet Program
Part One: The "Get Clean" Program
In gathering information on intestinal disorders, I read and extrapolated some of my written information from the research of the Journal of Current Gastroenterology Reports published by Current Medicine Group LLC, ISSN # 1522-8037 (Print), Volume 1, Number 5/October, 1999, DOI# 10.1007/s11894-999-0023-5, Pages 410-416, SpringerLink Date: May 23, 2007

For pH quotes see *The pH doc.,* publication *The pH Factor*-A REAL Silent Killer by Lyle Loughry, March 2007. The *Get Lean* quote by Dr. Richard Anderson was taken from *Cleanse & Purify Thyself.*

For more information on fasting and "eating to live," refer to Joel Fuhrman, M.D.'s book, *Fasting and Eating for Health: A Medical Doctor's Program for Conquering Disease.* Dr. Fuhrman's website is: www.drfuhrman.com

The definition of mucoid plaque which was coined by Dr. Richard Anderson was taken from the Wikipedia Encyclopedia at http://en.wikipedia.org/wiki/Mucoid/plaque.

Candida research was most taken from oncologist Dr. Simoncini in his book *Cancer is a*

Fungus. The spittle test can be found at: http://cassia.org/candiscussion.htm

Appetite Magazine, November 2007 edition quotes the Penn State University study regarding people who start a meal with vegetable soup ended up eating 20% less than those who skipped the soup.

Cruciferous vegetables known to activate liver enzymes responsible for clearing mercury; Williams, A.C., Steventon, G.B., et al., "Hereditary variation of liver enzymes involved with detoxification and neurodegenerative diseases." Journal of Inherited Metabolic Disorders 1991, Vol. 14: pp 431-435.

Chapter Ten: The EcoDiet Cook

For more information on conscious cooking and how cooking food at high temperatures creates digestive leukocytosis, refer to Premier Research Laboratories, Austin, Texas, an internationally preeminent manufacturer of premier quality nutraceutical formulations and superfood concentrates at http://www.prlabs.com

For more information on the hierarchy of food and food preparation, refer to Optimal Health Systems, Pima, Arizona, at www.optimalhealthsystems.com

RESOURCE SECTION

Organic-Biodynamic Produce

Whitted Bowers Fruit Farm
8707 Art Road
Cedar Grove, North Carolina 27231
1-919-732-5132
www.whittedbowersfarm@mac.com

Diamond Organics
The Organic Food Catalog
P.O. Box 2159
Freedom, California 95019
1-888-674-2642
www.diamondorganics.com

Farm Fresh To You
23808 State Highway 16
Capay, California 95607
1-800-796-6009
www.farmfreshtoyou.com

Ocean Grown, Inc.
7453 Commercial Circle
Ft. Pierce, Florida 34951
1-941-921-2401
www.oceangrown.com

Community Support Agriculture (CSA)
7200 Wisconsin Avenue
Suite 601
Bethesda, Maryland 20814
1-800-843-7751
www.csa.com

Organic Raw Foods, Supplements & Superfoods

Jaffe Brothers
28560 Lilac Road
Valley Center, California 92082
1-760-749-1133

UliMana, Inc.
P.O. Box 18058
Asheville, North Carolina 28814
1-828-713-3469
www.ulimana.com

Sunfood Nutrition
11655 Riverside Drive
Lakeside, California 92040
1-800-205-2350
www.sunfood.com

Sun Organic Farm
P.O. Box 409
San Marcos, California 92079
1-888-269-9888
www.sunorganic.com

Wilderness Family Naturals
1-800-945-3801
www.wildernessfamilynaturals.com

Great American Wholefood Farmacy
117 E. Main Street
Rogersville, Tennessee 37857
1-423-921-7848
www.wholefoodfarmacy.com

Udo's Oil Blends
Found at most health food stores
www.udoerasmus.com

Celtic Sea Salt®
Selina Naturally
4 Celtic Drive, Arden NC 28704
1-800-867-7258

Living Qi Organic Matcha Green Tea
Living Qi LLC
1-877-544-2583
www.living-qi.com

Active Manuka Honey & Royal Jelly
CalComp Nutrition Inc.
2021 Clay Pike, Suite 1
Irwin, PA 15642
1-877-919-9992

Rice Bran Complex
"Genesis Complex"
Lifestar
P. O. Box 3837
Sedona, AR 86340
1-877-793-4191

Matt Monarch
www.therawfoodworld.com

Paul Nison
www.rawlifee.com

Arise & Shine
Richard Anderson, N.D.
562 Parsons Drive
Medford, Oregon 97501
1-800-688-2444
www.ariseandshine.com

Morter Health Systems
215 West Poplar
Rogers, Arkansas 72756
1-800-874-1478
www.morterhealthsystem.com

The Synergy Company
2279 South Resource Boulevard
Moab, Utah 84532
1-800-723-0277
www.thesynergycompany.com

Sun Warrior Superfoods
www.getcleangogreenecodiet.com

Sun Chlorella
3305 Kashiwa Street
Torrance, California 90505
1-800-829-2828
www.sunchlorella.com

Nature's Balance Chlorella
913 Finch Avenue
High Point, North Carolina 27263
1-800-858-5198
www.natures-balance.com

Hallelujah Acres
900 S. Post Road
Shelby, North Carolina 28152
1-704-481-1700
www.hacres.com

Synergistic Nutrition
Stephen Heuer
1-864-895-6250
www.sgn80.com

Quantum Light Nutrition
Dr. Bob Marshall
19227 Pleasant Valley Road
North San Juan, California 95960
1-888-303-3004
www.quantumlightnutrition.com

Health Force Nutritionals
1835A S. Centre City Pkwy. #411
Escondido, California 92025
1-800-357-2717
www.healthforce.com

Enzymes & Liquid Oxygen

Natural Choice Products
109 Cooperative Way, Suite #101
Kalispell, Montana 59901
1-800-626-5143

Transformation Enzymes
2900 Wilcrest Drive #220
Houston, Texas 77042
1-713-266-2117
www.transformationenzymes.com

Intestinal Cleansing & Probiotics

Arise & Shine
Richard Anderson, ND
562 Parsons Drive
Medford, Oregon 97501
1-800-688-2444
www.ariseandshine.com

Christopher Herbs
Dr. John Christopher
155 West 2050 N.
Spanish Fork, Utah 84660
1-800-453-1406

V. E. Irons
1-800-544-8147
P.O. Box 34710
North Kansas City, MO 64116
www.veirons.com

Ejuva
2117 Timneh Court
Oceanside, CA 92057
1-866-463-5882
www.ejuva.com

The Alkalizer
Arise & Shine
562 Parsons Drive, Suite 110
1-800-688-2444
www.ariseandshine.com

Flora Grow Probiotics
Arise & Shine
562 Parsons Drive, Suite 110
1-800-688-2444
www.ariseandshine.com

Dr. Ohhira's Probiotics
Professional Formula
www.iherb.com

Candida, Parasites & Heavy Metal Detox

Organic Colloidal Silver &
Grapefruit Seed Extract
Arise & Shine
562 Parsons Drive, Suite 110
1-800-688-2444
www.getcleangogreenecodiet.com

EcoDiet Kitchen Equipment

Breville Juicer
www.getcleangogreenecodiet.com

BlendTec
www.getcleangogreenecodiet.com

Excalibur Dehydrators
www.getcleangogreenecodiet.com

Ionized Alkaline Water
www.getcleangogreenecodiet.com

AutoSprout
www.heartlandautosprout.com

Holistic Healing Clinics

Optimum Health Institute
6970 Central Avenue
Lemon Grove, California 91945
1-800-993-4325
www.optimumhealth.org

Hippocrates Health Institute
1443 Palmdale Court
West Palm Beach, Florida 33411
1-800-842-2125
www.hippocratesinst.org

Lorne Label, MD
Brain Longevity Center
2100 Lynn Road, Suite 230
Thousand Oaks, California 91360
1-805-497-4500
www.cns-neurology.com

Tree of Life Rejuvenation Center
Gabriel Cousens, MD
P.O. Box 778
Patagonia, Arizona 85624
1-866-394-2520
www.treeoflife.nu

Alternative Cancer Clinic
Saint Joseph Medical Center
Dr. Rogers and Dr. Rayes
www.doctorofhope.com

Jerry Tennant, MD
Tennant Institute for Integrative Medicine
9901 East Valley Ranch Parkway, #1015
Irving, Texas 75063
1-866-612-4461
www.tennantinstitute.com

Dave Carpenter, ND
Path To Health
Idaho Falls, Idaho
1-208-529-0384
www.pathtohealth.com

Thomas Rau, MD
Paracelsus Biological Clinic
c/o The Marion Institute
3 Barnabas Road
Marion, Massachusetts 02738
1-508-748-0816

Holistic Denistry

Darick Nordstrom, DDS
930 Sunnyslope Road, Suite D4
Hollister, CA 95023
1-831-637-1675

Robert Chan, DDS
Suite 11, 2425 East Street
Concord, CA 94520-1926
1-925-363-3902

Raymond Silkman, DDS
11645 Wilshire Boulevard
Brentwood, CA 90025
1-310-445-9098

Glen Sperbeck, DDS
6206 West 87th Street
Westhester, CA 90045
1-310-670-6944

Phil David, DDS
655 Brevard Road
Asheville, North Carolina 28806
1-828-670-9394

Colon Cleansing & Rejuvenation Center

Angel Farms
Cindy Sellers
www.angelfarms.com

Custom Nutrition and Blood Testing

American Metabolic Testing Laboratory
Emile Schandle, Ph.D.
1818 Sheridan Street #102
Hollywood, Florida 33020
1-954-929-4814

Forgiveness and Emotional Healing

HeartLand Teaching Center
Dr. Michael Ryce
Theodosia, Missouri 65761
1-417-273-4838
www.Iforgive.net

Energetic Clearing Process
Judith Johnson
329 Eden Drive
Hillsborough, North Carolina
1-919-241-3151
www.energeticclearingprocess.com

Rebirthing Breathwork
Leonard Orr, Rebirther
P.O. Box 1026
Staunton, Virginia 24404
1-540-885-0551
www.rebirthingbreathwork.com

Rebirthing Breathwork
Sondra Ray, Rebirther
www.sondraray.com

Rebirthing Breathwork
Steve Clymer, Rebirther
5901 Hollywood Blvd.
Sarasota, Florida 34231
1-941-921-5330
www.stevenclymer.com

Recommended Reading

Cleanse & Purify Thyself
Author: Dr. Richard Anderson
P.O. Box 1643
Medford, Oregon 97501
1-800-688-2444

Cancer is a Fungus
Author: Dr. Tullio Simoncini
www.cancerisafungus.com

The Germ that Causes Cancer
Author: Doug Kaufmann
www.knowthecause.com

Superfoods:
The Food & Medicine of the Future
Author: David Wolfe

Your Health Your Choice
Author: Dr. Ted Morter, Jr.
215 West Poplar
Rogers, Arkansas 72756
1-800-874.-478
www.morter.com

The China Study
Author T. Colin Campbell
www.thechinastudy.com

Healing is Voltage
Author: Jerry Tennant, MD
9901 East Valley Ranch Parkway, #1015
Irving, Texas 75063
1-866-612-4461
www.tennantinstitute.com

Farmacist Desk Reference
Author: Don Tolman
www.dontolman.com

Alkalize or Die
Author: Dr. Ted Baroody
119 Pigeon Street
Waynesville, North Carolina 28786
1-800-566-1522
www.holographichealth.com

The Swiss Secret to Optimal Health
Author: Dr. Thomas Rau, MD
Paracelsus Biological Medicine Network
c/o The Marion Institute
3 Barnabas Road
Marion, Massachusetts 02738
1-508-748-0816

Michael F. Holick, MD
Author: The UV Advantage
715 Albany Street M-1013
Boston, MA 02118
1-617-638-4545

Why is this Happening to me AGAIN?
Author: Dr. Michael Ryce
Route 3; Box 3280
Theodosia, Missouri 65761
1-417-273-4838
www.whyagain.com

The Biology of Belief
Author: Bruce Lipton, Ph.D.
www.brucelipton.com

Spontaneous Evolution
Authors: Bruce Lipton, Ph.D.
Steve Bhaerman
www.wakeuplaughing.com

The Secret
1235-A North Clybourn Avenue
Chicago, Illinois 60610
www.thesecret.tv

The Curse of Louis Pasteur
Author: Nancy Appleton, Ph.D.
P.O. Box 3083
Santa Monica, California 90403
www.nancyappleton.com

Conscious Language
Author: Robert Tennyson Stevens
352 Depot Street, Suite 210
Asheville, North Carolina 28801
1-828-258-2220
www.masterysystems.com

My Big Toe
Thomas Campbell
www.mybigtoe.com

Green for Life
Author: Victoria Boutenko
The Raw Family
Ashland, Oregon 975520
www.rawfamily.com

Breathing: The Master Key to Self Healing
Author: Andrew Weil, MD
www.drweil.com

Rainbow Green Live-Food Cuisine
Author: Gabriel Cousens, MD
Tree of Life Rejuvenation Center
P.O. Box 778
Patagonia, Arizona 85624
1-866-394-2520
www.treeoflife.nu

The Food Revolution
Author: John Robbins
www.foodrevolution.org

The Power of Your Plate
Author: Neal Barnard, MD
www.nealbarnard.org

Organic Clothes
Maggie's Organics
1-800-609-8593
www.maggiesorganics.com

Foundations To Support

Physicians Committee for Responsible
Medicine
5100 Wisconsin Ave., N.W., Suite 400
Washington, DC 20016
1-202-686-2210
www.pcrm.org

Earth Save Foundation
20555 Devonshire Blvd.
Suite #105
Chatsworth, CA 91311
1-818-407-0289

Positive World Enterprises
New York, New York
www.thinkpositiveamerica.com

INDEX